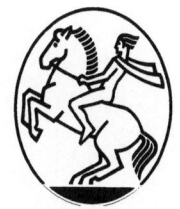

Neurotraumatology: Progress and Perspectives

Proceedings of the International Conference
on Recent Advances in Neurotraumatology,
Porto (Portugal), November 1990

Edited by
A. Martins da Silva, A. Rocha Melo,
F. Loew

Acta Neurochirurgica
Supplementum 55

Springer-Verlag Wien New York

Professor Dr. A. Martins da Silva
Department of Neurophysiology, Hospital Santo Antonio, Porto, and
Unit of Human Physiology, Biomedical Institute "Abel Salazar", University of Porto, Portugal

Professor Dr. A. Rocha Melo
Department of Neurosurgery, Hospital Santo Antonio, Porto, Portugal

Professor Dr. F. Loew
Neurochirurgische Universitätsklinik, Homburg/Saar, Federal Republic of Germany

With 34 Figures

ISSN 0065-1419
ISBN-13: 978-3-7091-9235-1   e-ISBN-13: 978-3-7091-9233-7
DOI: 10.1007/978-3-7091-9233-7

Preface

Neurotraumatology: Progresses and Perspectives summarize the interventions of experts, from neurotraumatology or other neurosciences to biophysics and bioengineering, during the ICRAN Meeting – International Conference on Recent Advances in Neurotraumatology – held in Porto, Portugal, in November 1990 and organized under the auspices of the Neurotraumatology Committee of the World Federation of Neurosurgical Societies. This Committee was the great promoter of the meeting, organized in Portugal for the first time. The organizers remembered and dedicated their work to the efforts developed by Dr. Vasconcellos Marques, Past-President of the Committee, in encouraging neurotrauma research.

Following the general principles of the *Acta Neurochirurgica*, the editors reviewed and selected the papers here included and presented to the meeting. The texts illustrate that the progresses in current neurotraumatology research result from the interaction of different disciplines. The discussion of the topics has been deep and multidisciplinary and based on new methods of imaging and of metabolic studies, new techniques for patient monitoring, advances in patient treatment with new drugs and progress in techniques of patient recovering processes. Final emphasis was given to the socioeconomic impact of head trauma accidents.

The impressive number of new cases of head trauma occurring each year as a result of civillian accidents – traffic, domestic and work – in industrialized countries gives sufficient data and highlights the understanding of brain functioning pathophysiology even in the case of ill-identified consequences. The fruitfull discussion during the meeting raised the outlines of new research fields and brought about further perspectives into the comprehension of the head trauma long-term consequences. This will enable the adoption of new strategies on patients rehabilitation, a better knowledge of the damaged brain pathophysiology, and the hope that new contributions may be given to patient recovery, thus minimizing the costs of this „severe epidemic of the industrialized world".

We would like to thank the Neurotrauma Committee for promoting this meeting, Dr. H. Gossman for his effort in reviewing the texts and Mrs. Amelia Santos for typing the manuscripts. We also thank Pharmaceutical Companies for their financial support and from the JNICT (Porguese Agency for Science and Technology) for rendering possible the organization of the meeting.

A. Martins da Silva
A. Rocha Melo

Contents

Acta Neurochir (1992) [Suppl] 55: 1–5

Evaluation of Intracranial Pressure Gradients by Means of Transcranial Doppler Sonography

E. R. Cardoso[1] and **J. A. Kupchak**[2]

[1] Cerebral Hydrodynamics Research Laboratory, [1,2] Departments of [1] Surgery and [2] Nursing Education and Research, Health Sciences Centre, Winnipeg, Manitoba, Canada

Summary

The authors investigated the effects of intracranial pressure gradients generated by a unilateral intracranial mass on transcranial Doppler (TCD) readings. Eleven patients harbouring a symptomatic chronic or subacute subdural haematoma underwent pre- and post-operative TCD examinations of the intracranial internal carotid and middle cerebral arteries. Mean values of velocity and pulsatility index (PI) were compared to the contra-lateral counterpart. The haematomas were evacuated by means of burr hole drainage under local anaesthesia.

Symptomatic subdural haematomas lowered the ipsilateral blood velocity in the internal carotid and middle cerebral arteries by a mean side-to-side difference of 15.64 ± 3.01 m.sec^{-1}. The ipsilateral PI was higher than the contralateral values by an average of 0.23 ± 0.04. Low mean velocity and high PI values were associated with high subdural pressure. Abnormal pre-operative ipsilateral TCD readings returned to normal following haematoma drainage.

We postulate that intracranial pressure gradients generated by the subdural mass lesion are responsible for the asymmetry of TCD readings. These differences should be considered in the interpretation of post-subarachnoid haemorrhage vasospasm, as it is frequently associated with lateral clots. Our findings also provide a useful method for non-invasive monitoring of intracranial pressure gradients.

Keywords: Head injury; intracranial pressure gradients; subdural haematoma; transcranial Doppler; sonography; ultrasound.

List of Abbreviations

CT = computerized tomography
GCS = Glasgow Coma Scale
ICP = intracranial pressure
NSD = no significant difference
PI = pulsatility index
SAH = subarachnoid hemorrhage
TCD = Transcranial Doppler

Introduction

Blood flow velocity depends on the vessel radius, the blood viscosity, and the pressure gradient between the two ends of the vessels considered. Changes of flow velocity induced by alterations of vascular radius, as in post-subarachnoid haemorrhage (SAH) vasospasm, have been extensively used in clinical practice[1, 2, 14, 15, 17, 18, 21]. Others have used transcranial Doppler (TCD) to evaluate cerebral vascular auto-regulation and pCO_2 response[3, 5, 22, 24]. However, the effects of elevated intracranial pressure (ICP) on TCD readings have not been fully studied. Investigators have examined the TCD changes produced by severe diffuse elevations of the ICP, but not the effects of focal ICP increases. Diffuse elevation of ICP lowers the cerebral perfusion pressure and the diastolic blood flow velocity through the major intracranial vessels, thus increasing the pulsatility index (PI)[13, 17, 19, 27, 28].

In order to investigate the effects of focal elevation of ICP on TCD readings we prospectively examined patients harbouring a unilateral hemispheric subdural haematoma by means of bilateral TCD examinations performed before and after haematoma drainage.

Material and Methods

Patient Population

Eleven consecutive patients with a subdural haematoma were evaluated, including 10 males and 1 female. Their mean age was 67.7 years, ranging from 39 to 86 years. All haematomas resulted from low velocity trauma. No patient had coagulopathy. All patients presented focal neurological findings attributable to the haematoma. The pre-operative mean GCS was 12, ranging from 8 to 15, while post-operatively it was 15 in all patients. The focal neurological deficits had disappeared in all patients the day after surgery.

This patient population allowed us to measure intra-operative subdural pressures without the interference of anesthesia or hyperventilation. To qualify several criteria had to be met: 1) presence of a single symptomatic subacute or chronic subdural haematoma, 2) presence of focal neurological findings attributable to the location of the haematoma, 3) satisfactory patient co-operation for performance of TCD readings and haematoma evacuation under local anaesthesia, and 4) no pre-treatment with steroids or diuretics. The haematomas had been diagnosed by computerized axial tomography (CT). The greatest CT midline shift of the septum pellucidum was measured in mm for correlation with TCD values of mean velocity and PI.

The TCD examinations were performed with a model TC 2-64B EME Transcranial Doppler machine, coupled with a 2 MHz. PW probe* just prior to surgical evacuation. TCD mean velocity and PI measurements of both the internal carotid and middle cerebral arteries were taken from the temporal windows, at depth settings of 65, 60, 55 and 50 mm, with patients in the supine position. The highest stable reading at each depth setting was selected. Values for the four depth settings were then averaged. This averaged figure was then compared to the contra-lateral counterpart. Pre- and post-operative examinations were always performed by the same examiner. Blood pressure measurements, Glasgow Coma Scale [GCS] scores and arterial pCO_2 values were recorded at the time of TCD readings.

Surgical evacuation of haematomas was carried out on awake patients in the supine position, through a single burr hole. Prior to drainage, a number 16 gauge curved needle was introduced into the subdural space through the intact dura matter and manometric measurement of the subdural pressure was recorded. The haematoma was then completely evacuated and the subdural space washed with warm saline solution. A draining catheter was left in the subdural space, externalized through a separate stab wound, and connected to a low-pressure suction device.

Post-operative measurements of subdural pressure, TCD velocities and PI were performed the day after surgery. Subdural pressure was reduced to zero by opening the distal end of the catheter to the atmosphere, just before TCD readings. Only patients with patent drains were selected for ascertaining that the post-operative subdural pressure was indeed zero. Post-operative blood pressure, GCS scores and arterial pCO_2 values were also recorded.

Statistical comparisons were made by means of two-tailed paired t-test. Variations from the mean are given as standard error.

Results

Pre-Operative Findings

TCD mean velocities were lower on the side of the subdural haematoma in all but one patient. The mean velocity on the side of the subdural haematoma was 34.18 ± 2.22 m.sec^{-1} and 49.2 ± 1.2 m.sec^{-1} on the contra-lateral side. The side-to-side difference of 15.64 ± 3.01 m.sec^{-1} was statistically significant (P < 0.0005) and correlated inversely with the patients age (R= –0.63).

Pre-operative PI measurements were greater on the side of the haematoma by a mean side-to-side difference of 0.23 ± 0.04 (P < 0.0025). The PI averaged 1.33 ± 0.01 on the side of the mass and 1.11 ± 0.05 on the contra-lateral side. Post-operatively, the ipsilateral PI was $1.08 + 0.01$ and contra-lateral PI 1.05 ± 0.06 (NSD) (Fig. 1).

Side-to-side differences of gated measurements taken

---

*EME 19226, 66th Ave. S., Kent, Washington, 98032 U.S.A.

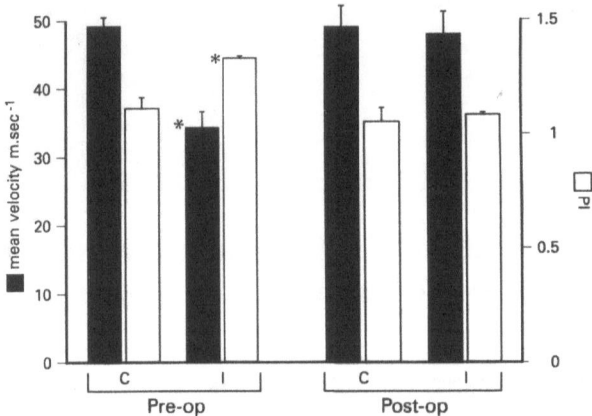

Fig. 1. Internal carotid and middle cerebral arteries transcranial Doppler mean blood flow velocities (black bars) and pulsatility index (PI) (white bars) for contralateral (C) and ipsilateral (I) readings. Pre-operatively, there were significant (*) side-to-side differences for mean velocities and PI. These differences disappeared after evacuation of haematomas (post-op)

at depth of 65 mm were compared to those taken at 50 mm depth. No significant difference was encountered, indicating that the subdural mass was affecting equally the flow velocities in the internal as well as midle cerebral arteries. There was poor correlation between the magnitude of midline shift on CT scan and the side-to-side differences of mean velocity and PI (R= –0.22 and –0.41). This observation is in agreement with the lack of correlation between size of midline shift and intracranial pressure values found by other investigators[12, 31].

Operative Findings

Intra-operative subdural pressure was measured in 8 patients. The manometer became plugged by old clotted blood in two, and subdural fluid leaked around the needle in another patient. The mean subdural pressure was 13.19 ± 2.93 cm H2O. Subdural pressures did not correlate with side-to-side differences of mean TCD velocities (R = 0.43), but correlated well with differences of mean PI (R = 0.85).

Post-Operative Findings

Following removal of the subdural haematoma the ipsilateral flow velocity increased significantly from 34.18 ± 2.22 m.sec^{-1} to 47.9 ± 3.2 m.sec^{-1} (P < 0.002) (Fig. 2).

On the contra-lateral side however, there was no significant difference between the mean pre- and post-operative values of 49.2 ± 1.2 m.sec^{-1} and 49.0 ± 3.0 m.sec^{-1} for mean flow velocities. Similarly, evacuation of the clot normalized ipsilateral PI values and elimi-

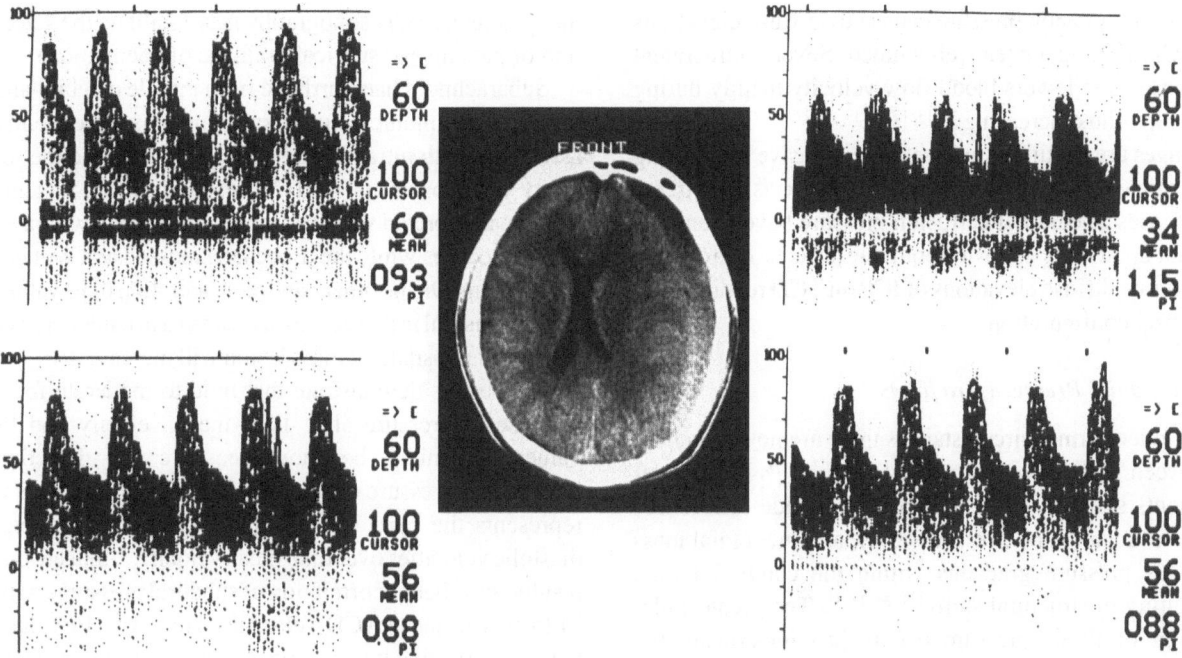

Fig. 2. Example of a representative patient harbouring a left chronic subdural haematoma. Top: Pre-operative TCD values taken at 60 mm depth setting, showing side-to-side differences of 26 cm.sec^{-1} for mean velocity and 0.22 for pulsatility index (PI). Bottom: Post-operative TCD tracings showing normalization of left sided TCD values and disappearance of side-to-side asymmetry

Table 1. *Doppler Blood Flow Velocity and Pulsality Index Before and After Subdural Haematomas Surgery*

	Pre-op		Post-op	
	ipsilateral	contralateral	ipsilateral	contralateral
Mean velocity (m/sec)	34.18 ± 2.22	49.2 ± 1.2*	47.9 ± 3.2	49.0 ± 3.0 +
PI	1.33 ± 0.01	1.11 ± 0.05**	1.08 ± 0.02	1.05 ± 0.06 +
Δ V (m/sec)	15.64 ± 3.01		2.55 ± 2.9	
Δ PI	0.23 ± 0.04		0.06 ± 0.1	

*P < 0.0005; **P < 0.0025; + NSD (not significant differences); PI = Pulsatility index.

nated pre-operative asymmetries. The mean pre-operative ipsilateral PI value of 1.33 ± 0.01 went down to 1.08 ± 0.01 (P < 0.01). The contra-lateral side showed no significant change from 1.11 ± 0.05 to 1.05 ± 0.06 (Table 1).

The alterations of TCD readings between pre- and post-operative measurements could not be attributed to changes of mean blood pressure or arterial pCO2 content, as they did not change significantly. Pre-operative values were 98.2 ± 28 mmHg and 35.0 ± 1.0 mmHg respectively, while the corresponding post-operative values were 98.6 ± 2.35 mmHg and 34.8 ± 1.0 mmHg.

Discussion

TCD is a non-invasive technique for the measurement of blood velocity in the major intra-cranial arteries[3, 16, 18, 21, 27]. According to the Hagen-Poiseuille's law, TCD readings depend upon the pressure gradient between the two ends of the vessel considered, its radius, and the viscosity of the circulating blood[8, 27, 32]. The effects of alterations of vascular radius on TCD readings have been extensively investigated in patients with post-SAH vasospasm[1, 2, 14, 17, 18, 21, 27]. Furthermore, the effects of diffuse reductions of cerebral perfusion pressure caused by diffuse elevations of ICP have also been well studied. Severe intracranial hypertension lowers blood flow velocity mainly during diastole, thus increasing PI[13, 15, 17, 19, 21, 27, 28]. These TCD changes are useful for indirect, non-invasive monitoring of critical elevation of ICP. While the effects of extreme decreases of cerebral perfusion pressure have been well defined, little is known about the effects of focal or moderate diffuse elevations of ICP on TCD readings and spectral configuration.

Intracranial Pressure Gradients

Under normal circumstances there are no differences between TCD values form side to side[3, 16, 28]. Indeed, our patients showed no significant side-to-side differences after evacuation of clots. However, an intracranial mass creates pressure gradients within the cerebral tissue, resulting in structural shifts[4, 9, 25, 26, 33]. The greatest elevation of tissue pressure occurs just underneath the subdural clot, and progressively decreases radially from the mass[4, 26]. Raised tissue pressure lowers intravascular blood flow velocity. Thus, we believe that in our cases the asymmetry of TCD readings was due to raised interstitial pressure underlying the subdural haematoma.

There was an inverse relationship between age and pre-operative TCD gradients, confirming previous evidence of a greater pressure effect by the mass in younger patients[6, 7, 11].

The possibility that our findings resulted from error introduced by poor transmission of echogenic signals through the subdural fluid has been ruled out on two accounts. Firstly, bloody fluids are good ultrasonic conductors, and while the amplitude of the signal was decreased the signal intensity was unchanged. TCD signal intensity reflects volume of circulating blood and velocity amplitude reflects speed of blood flow. Secondly, low ipsilateral TCD velocity and high PI were also observed with intracerebral haematomas and brain tumours.

Possible Clinical Applications

Our results suggest future applications for the use of TCD sonography in: 1) the prediction of impending cerebral herniation with lateral mass lesions, 2) better assessment of results in patients with cerebral vasospasm and associated intracerebral clots, and 3) the evaluation of moderate elevations of intracranial pressure.

Selection of patients for surgical removal of some intracranial haematomas remains controversial as many patients respond to conservative treatment[12, 23, 31]. Thus, in these patients, TCD sonography may facilitate the selection of patients for surgical drainage of haematomas.

Subarachnoid haemorrhage from middle cerebral and posterior communicating artery aneurysms is frequently associated with intracerebral clots, wich increase the severity of vasospasm[10, 20]. TCD results in these patients must be interpreted with caution, as vasospasm will raise TCD velocities while the associated mass lesion will decrease them. On the other hand, consideration of PI values becomes useful in these cases, as vasospasm tends to lower PI, while an ipsilateral mass lesion will increase it.

Our results demonstrate that mild to moderate focal increase in pressure alter TCD mean velocity and PI values. PI might be more sensitive for detecting intracranial pressure changes than mean velocities, as it represents the ratio between peak systolic minus end diastolic velocities over time mean velocity[21]. Indeed, our results show better correlation of subdural pressures with PI than with mean TCD velocities. However, PI values have not received the same attention as mean TCD velocities in the literature[15, 27]. Furthermore, future studies are needed to ascertain whether diffuse elevations of intracranial pressure of the same magnitude will produce similar changes of PI and mean TCD velocities.

Sequential TCD readings post-evacuation of a subdural mass can be used as an inexpensive and non-invasive method for investigating the possibility of haematoma re-accumulation. Future studies are required to establish whether the magnitude of difference between TCD readings from both sides could determine which haematomas require surgical evacuation or conservative treatment[19, 30].

Acknowledgements

The authors are indebted to the Grand Lodge of Free Masons of Manitoba, the Head Injury Association of Manitoba and the Children's Hospital Association for financial support of this project. We also thank Dr. M. R. Del Bigio for critical review of the manuscript.

References

1. Aaslid R, Huber P, Normes H (1984) Evaluation of cerebrovascular spasm with transcranial Doppler ultrasound. J Neurosurg 60: 37–41
2. Aaslid R, Huber P, Nornes H (1986) A transcranial Doppler method in evaluation of cerebrovascular spasm. Neuroradiology 28: 11–16
3. Aaslid R, Markwalder T, Normes H (1982) Non-invasive transcranial Doppler ultrasound recording of flow velocity in basal cerebral arteries. J Neurosurg 57: 769–774
4. Abe T, Black PM, Foley L (1984) Changes in parenchymal and ventricular pressure with experimental epidural compression. Surg Neurol 22: 477–480

5. Bishop CC, Powell S, Insall M, *et al* (1986) Effect of internal carotid artery occlusion on middle cerebral artery blood flow at rest and in response to hypercapnia. Lancet – March: 710–712

6. Cardoso ER, Del Bigio MR, Schroeder G (1989) Age-dependent changes of cerebral ventricular size. Part I: review of intracranial fluid collections. Acta Neurochir (Wien) 97: 40–46

7. Cardoso ER, Del Bigio MR (1989) Age-related changes of cerebral ventricular size. Part II: normalization of ventricular size following shunting. Acta Neurochir (Wien) 97: 135–138

8. Delin NA, Ekestrom S, Telenius R (1968) Relation of degree of internal carotid artery stenosis to blood flow and pressure gradient. An angiographic and surgical study in man. Invest Radiol 3: 337–334

9. Findlay GF, Cummings BH (1981) Contralateral ventricular dilatation in supratentorial tumors. J Neurosurg 54: 509–512

10. Fisher CM, Kistler PJ, Davis JM (1980) Relation of cerebral vasospasm to subarachnoid hemorrhage visualized by computed tomographic scanning. Neurosurgery 6: 1–9

11. Fogelholm R, Heiskanen O, Waltimo O (1975)Chronic subdural hematomas in adults. J Neurosurg 42: 43–46

12. Galbraith S, Teasdale G (1981) Predicting the need for operation in the patient with an occult traumatic intracranial hematoma. J Neurosurg 55: 77–81

13. Glawloski J, Hassler W (1989) Significance of transcranial doppler sonography in cerebral injury: influence of hemodynamic changes on therapeutic management. Neurosurg Rev 12: 386–388

14. Gilsbach JM, Harders A (1985) Early aneurysm operation and vasospasm-intracranial Doppler findings. Neurochirurgia 28: 100–103

15. Giulioni M, Ursino M, Alvisi C (1988) Correlations among intracranial pulsatility; intracranial hemodynamics and transcranial Doppler wave form. Literature review and hypothesis for future studies. Neurosurgery 22–5: 807–811

16. Grolimund P. Seiler RW, Aaslid R, *et al* (1987) Evaluation of cerebrovascular disease by combined extracranial and transcranial Doppler sonography. Stroke 18: 1018–1024

17. Grote E, Hassler W (1988) The critical first minutes after subarachnoid hemorrhage. Neurosurg 22–4: 654–661

18. Harders A, Gilsbach JM (1987) Time cours of blood velocity related to vasospasm in the circle of Willis measured by transcranial Doppler ultrasound. J Neurosurgery 66: 718–728

19. Hassler W, Steinmetz H, Gawlowski J (1988) Transcranial Doppler ultrasonography in raised intracranial pressure and in intracranial circulatory arrest. J Neurosurg 68: 745–751

20. Kistler JP, Crowell RM, Davies KR, *et al* (1983) The relation of cerebral vasospasm to the extent and location of subarachnoid blood visualizad by CT scan: a prospective study. Neurology 33: 424–436

21. Lindegaard K, Bakke SJ, Gromilund P, *et al* (1985) Assessment of intracranial hemodynamics in carotid artery disease by transcranial Doppler ultrasound. J Neurosurg 63: 890–898

22. Lundar T, Lindegaard K, Froysaker T, *et al* (1985) Dissociation between cerebral autoregulation and CO2 reactivity during nonpulsatile cardiopulmonary bypass. Ann Thorac Surg 40–6: 582–587

23. Markwalder T–M (1981) Chronic subdural hematomas: a review. Neurosurgery 54: 637–645

24. Markwalder T, Grolimund P, Seiler R, *et al* (1984) Dependency of blood flow velocity in the middle cerebral artery on end-tidal carbon dioxide partial pressure – a transcranial ultrasound doppler study. J Cereb Blood Flow Metabol 4: 368–372

25. Marmarou A, Poll W, Shapiro K, *et al* (1976) Time course of brain tissue pressure and compartmental CSF pressure in cerebral edema. Sug Forum 27: 483–485

26. Penn RD, Bacus JW (1984) The brain as a sponge: a computed tomographic look at Hakim's hypothesis. Neurosurgery 14: 670–675

27. Ringelstein EB (1986) Transcranial Doppler monitoring. In: Aaslid R (ed) Transcranial Doppler sonography. Springer, Wien, New York, pp 147–161

28. Shigemori M, Nakashima H, Moriyama T, *et al* (1989) Noninvasive study of critical thresholds of intracranial pressure and cerebral perfusion pressure for cerebral circulation and brain function. Neurol Res 11: 165–168

29. Suzuki J, Takaku A (1970) Nonsurgical treatment of chronic subdural hematoma. J Neurosurg 33: 548–553

30. Takeuchi T, Tsubokawa T, Hauashi N, *et al* (1988) Prognosis of chronic subdural hematoma using non-invasive skull impendance plethysmography. Neurol Med Chir 28: 654–660

31. Teasdale G, Galbraith S, Jennett B (1980) Operate or observe? ICP and the management of the "silent" traumatic intracranial hematoma. In: Shulman K, Marmarou A, Miller JD, *et al* (eds) Intracranial Pressure IV. Springer, Berlin Heidelberg New York, pp 36–38

32. Toole JF, Patel AN (1967) Cerebrovascular Disorders. McGraw-Hill, Toronto, pp 65–69

33. Weaver DD, Winn HR, Jane JA (1982) Differential intracranial pressure in patients with unilateral mass lesions. J Neurosurg 56: 660–665

Correspondence: Dr. Erico R. Cardoso, Director, Cerebral Hydrodynamics Research Laboratory, MS-767, Health Sciences Centre, 820 Sherbrook Street, Winnipeg, Manitoba, Canada R3C 1R9.

Acta Neurochir (1992) [Suppl] 55: 6–7

Monitoring of Severe Head-Injured Patients with Transcranial Doppler (TCD) Ultrasonography

M. Shigemori, N. Kikuchi, T. Tokutomi, S. Ochiai, K. Harada, T. Kikuchi, and **S. Kuramoto**

Department of Neurosurgery, Kurume University School of Medicine, Kurume, Japan

Summary

Intracranial haemodynamics were studied in 36 patients with severe head injury and experimental animals with acute intracranial hypertension by the use of TCD ultrasound. The mean flow velocity (FV) in the basal cerebral arteries commoly decreased on the side of the haematoma depending on intracranial pressure (ICP) elevation and cerebral perfusion pressure (CPP) reduction in focal brain injury. The FV decreased bilaterally and there was no difference between the right and left sides in diffuse brain injury without a clear relationship between the FV and CPP. The FV of the middle cerebral artery and blood flow in the internal carotid artery exhibited flow patterns which changed correlatively depending on CPP reduction in experimental animals. Monitoring with TCD ultrasound is valuable in evaluating compression ischaemia in focal brain injury. But many complicated factors are considerable in diffuse brain injury.

Keywords: Severe head injury; haemodynamic; ICP; TCD.

Introduction

Head-injured patients have been discussed by classifing their lesion types into diffuse and focal brain injury. One of the potential mechanism of brain damage in these patients is brain ischaemia secondary to intracranial hypertension[2, 3]. To clarify the different features of intracranial haemodynamics in diffuse and focal brain injury, we studied 36 patients with severe head injury and experimental animals with acute intracranial hypertension by use of transcranial Doppler (TCD) ultrasound[1].

Materials and Methods

We studied 36 patients including 16 with diffuse and 20 with focal brain injuries whose Glasgow Coma Scale (GCS) scores were 8 or less on admission. The age of the patients ranged from 5 to 78 years, with mean age of 38 years. The mean blood flow velocity (FV) in the basal cerebral arteries (M1, A1, P1, portions) were recorded using TCD ultrasound (TC 2-64 and transcran, EME) under end-tidal CO_2 monitoring. The pulsatility amplitude between the systolic and diastolic flow velocities (S/D ratio) was also recorded. Intracranial pressure (ICP) and systemic arterial blood pressure were also monitored to calculate cerebral perfusion pressure (CPP). Acute intracranial hypertension was produced by extradural balloon inflation in 10 monkeys (Macaca Fuscata) in order to determnine the correlation between the FV in the middle cerebral artery and blood flow in the internal carotid artery (ICBF) by use of TCD and electromagnetic flow meter (MFV 1100, Nihon Khoden).

Results

The FV in the bilateral basal cerebral arteries in patients with diffuse brain injury commonly decreased on admission and there was no significant difference between the right and the left sides. The FVs in the M1 and A1 portions increased transiently within 10 days after injury in patients with diffuse axonal injury, massive subarachnoid haemorrhage and diffuse cerebral swelling. There was no significant change in the S/D ratios in the basal cerebral arteries. But the FVs on the side of haematoma were commonly lower than those on the contralateral side in patients with focal brain injury. The S/D ratios were also commonly high on the side of haematoma. The FV in focal brain injury decreased depending on CPP reduction. But there was no correlation between them in patients with diffuse brain injury (Table 1).

The S/D ratios in the basal cerebral arteries also increased correlatively with CPP reduction in focal brain injury. On the relationship between the FV in the middle cerebral artery and CPP in experimental animals, the FV decreased with the ICBF and it decreased significantly when ICBF reduced to 70% or less compared to that before balloon inflation (Fig. 1).

Table 1. *Cerebral Perfusion Pressure (CCP) and MCA – Flow Velocity (MCA – FV)*

CPP (mmHg)	MCA – FV (cm/s)	
	diffuse brain injury (n: 33)	focal brain injury (n: 50)
40 or less	85.0 ± 26	44.1 ± 16*
41 ~ 60	91.0 ± 47	65.2 ± 31
61 ~ 80	118.0 ± 52*	74.5 ± 24
81 or more	68.5 ± 28	78.7 ± 27

* $P < 0.05$.

Control of MCA – FV: 67.0 ± 13 cm/s.

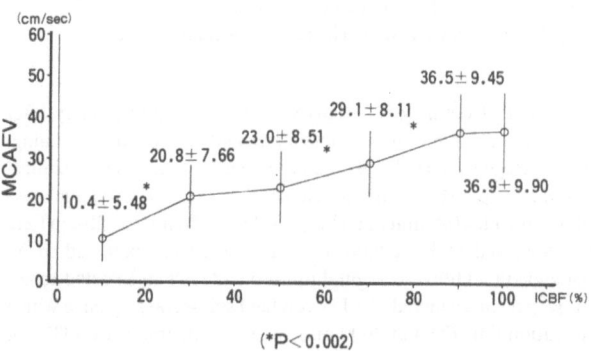

ICBF : internal carotid artery blood flow
MCAFV : middle cerebral artery mean flow velocity

Fig. 1. Relationship between MCAFV and ICBF (%)

Discussion

TCD ultrasound has now been widely used in the detection of intracranial haemodynamic phenomena because of its atraumatic and repeatable nature[1]. Although many complicated factors influence the intracranial blood flow velocities, a good correlation between the FV in the middle cerebral artery and ICBF was found in experimental animals with focal compression. Intracranial haematoma produces an increase of the ICP which caused compression of the cerebral veins, increased cerebrovascular resistance and decrease of cerebral blood flow. The present result in focal brain injury may therefore represent compression ischaemia in the hemisphere due to increased vascular resistance. The FV decreased significantly when CPP decreased to 40 mmHg or less. This may indicate their theresholds for cerebral circulatoroy disturbance in these patients[4]. In patients with diffuse brain injury, however, haemodynamic events are more complex than those in focal brain injury[2, 3]. Decreased FV in diffuse brain injury may indicate reduced cerebral blood flow commensurate with the reduction in global metabolic requirement due to diffusely damaged neurons[3]. It is known that cerebral blood flow is diffusely increased in patients with diffuse cerebral swelling[2] and traumatic subarachnoid haemorrhage often associated with narrowing of the caliber of the basal arteries[5]. Therefore many complicated factors other than ischaemia are pertinent in the interpretation of TCD data in patients with diffuse brain injury. But the monitoring with TCD can provide valuable information in evaluating different features of intracranial haemodynamics in severely head injured patients.

References

1. Aaslid R, Markwalder TM, Nores H (1982) Noninvasive transcranial Doppler ultrasound recording of flow velocity in basal cerebral arteries. J Neurosurg 57: 769–774
2. Miller JD (1982) Disorders of cerebral blood flow and intracranial pressure after head injury. Clin Neurosurg 29: 162–173
3. Obrist WD, Langfitt TW, Jaggi JL, Cruz J, Gennarelli TA (1984) Cerebral blood flow and metabolism in comatose patients with acute head injury. J Neurosurg 61: 241–253
4. Shigemori M, Nakashima H, Moriyama T, Tokutomi T, Nishio N, Harada K, Kuramoto S (1989) Noninvasive study of critical theresholds of intracranial pressure (ICP) and cerebral perfusion pressure (CPP) for cerebral circulation and brain function. Neurol Res 11: 165–168
5. Shigemori M, Tokutomi T, Hirohata M, Maruiwa H, Kaku N, Kuramoto S (1990) Clinical significance of traumatic subaracnoid hemorrhage. Neurol Med Chir (Tokyo 30: 396–400

Correspondence: Minoru Shigemori, M. D., Department of Neurosurgery, Kurume University School of Medicine, 67, Asahimachi, Kurume, 830, Japan.

Acta Neurochir (1992) [Suppl] 55: 8–10

Comparative Study of Magnetic Resonance and CT Scan Imaging in Cases of Severe Head Injury

T. Ogawa[1], H. Sekino[2], M. Uzura[2], T. Sakamoto[2], Y. Taguchi[2], Y. Yamaguchi[2], T. Hayashi[2], I. Yamanaka[3], N. Oohama[3], and S. Imaki[3]

[1] Division of Neurosurgery, [2] Department of Neurosurgery, St. Marianna University School of Medicine, Yokohama,
[3] Division of Emergency and Critical Care Medicine, St. Mariana University Yokohama City Seibu Hospital, Yokohama, Japan

Summary

The distribution, frequency, and appearance of head injuries were evaluated with MRI and CT in a prospective study of 155 patients with acute (n = 124) and chronic (n = 31) head injuries. MRI was significantly more sensitive than CT in the detection of intra-axial injury at any stage. In severe cases, central structure lesions were detected in approximately 80% of patients. Severity on admission was compatible with MR findings.

However it was difficult to decide on neurobehavioural prognosis from initial MRI findings only.

Keywords: Head injury; central structure; MR (Magnetic Resonance) imaging.

Introduction

Recently Magnetic Resonance (MR) Imaging is used to evaluate head injuries. It revealed lesions in more detail than computed tomography (CT) scan[2, 3]. We compared MRI vs CT scan concerning head injured patients, especially in the acute stage.

Materials and Methods

From July 1987 to August 1990, at St. Marianna University Yokohama City Seibu Hospital, neurological evaluation and morphological assessment using MRI and CT was performed in unselected head injury patients. Of 155 patients, 114 were males and 41 females. Age ranged from 3–78 years old. Infants and chronic subdural haematoma cases were excluded. Most cases were victims of road traffic accidents. Seventy-two severe cranial injury patients were the main focus of this study. Severe injury group included those with a score of under 8 on the Glasgow Coma Scale (GCS), moderate injury consisted of those with a score of 9–12 and the minor injury group consisted of those with GCS score of 13–15 on admission. The moderate group consisted of 76, and there were 6 in the minor head injury group. In acute severe cases, excluding operative treatment, mechanical ventilation was introduced conventionally.

High-resolution CT (Toshiba TCT900S) and MR (1.5T Philips) were used. Routinely CT scans were obtained immediately after admission using 8-mm thickness slices and contiguous sectioning. The average time for CT examination was 2–5 min. The technical parameters for MR include a field strength of 1.5 T, slice thickness of 5 mm with a 0.5-mm interslicegap, 256×256 matrix, 20-cm field of view, and two excitations. Axial scans were obtained in all patients, in addition to sagittal or coronal views in selected cases. Pulse sequences included a T2-weighted spin-echo sequence with a repetition time (TR) of 2000 msec and asymmetric echos (TEs) of 100, and a T1-weighted spin-echo sequence with TR = 460–1000 msec and TE = 20 msec. Average needed time for MR was 45 min.

For ease of lesion description term "central structure" includes corpus callosum, brainstem (midbrain, pons and medulla), cingulate gyrus, basal ganglia, and septal area.

Results

Superior sensitivity of MR was recognized in the evaluation of the site and size of the lesions (Table 1).

In general extra-axial lesions assessment is almost the same. However concerning intra-axial lesions and central structures, sensitivity could be twice to five times superior depending on the site MRI was recognized.

In the minor head injury group, small contusions of the temporal tip or frontal base were noted on MRI but they could not be verified by CT. In the moderate group multiplicity of cortical injury was characteristic on MR. In the severe injury group, all but one lesion was detected, and especially central structure injury was revealed by MRI.

Especially on "pure perimesencephalic SAH findings on CT" cases, MRI disclosed an accompanying corpus callosum lesion in half of the cases. Distribution of corpus callosum injury was demonstrable only in the sagittal plane (Fig. 1, 2).

Clinically so-called diffuse axonal injury (DAI) cases showed wide difference in MR findings. There was no

Table 1. *MRI and CT Assessment of Head Injury. Detected Lesions and Number by MR vs CT on 108 Cases*

	MR	CT	superiority
Extraaxial			same
epidural*	28	32	
subdural*	19	37	
subarachnoid	5	19	
Cortex	83	58	MR
Subcortical region (inc. corona radiata)	32	22	MR
Central structures	49	11	MR
corpus callosum	19	6	
septal area (inc.fornix)	6	2	
cingulate gyrus (inc.hippocamp.)	9	3	
basal ganglia	12	5	
midbrain	6	0	
pons	3	0	
Cerebellum	18	5	MR
Total	256	178	
Extraaxial*			
fracture			CT?
air / air cell			
CSDH	62	62	same?
hygroma	6	5	same?

* Including operated case.

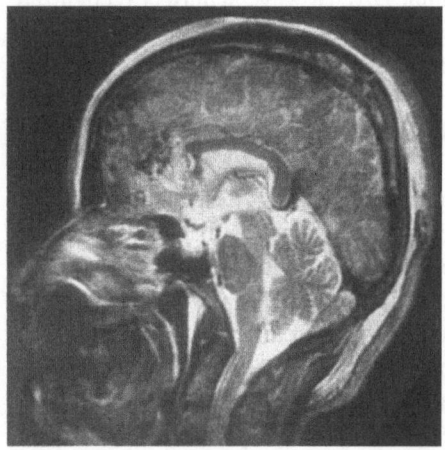

Fig. 1. A-51-year-old woman with callosal and septal area injury suffered long term aphasia but recovered finally

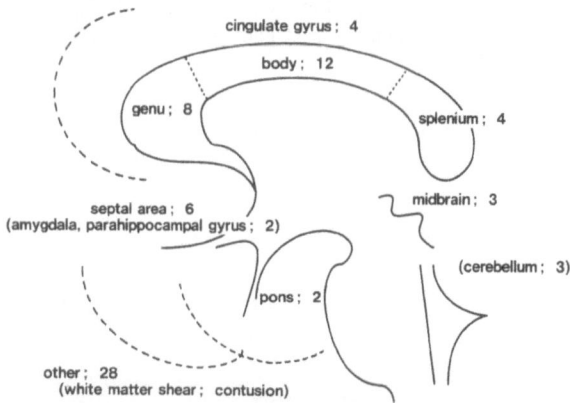

Fig. 2. Distribution of corpus callosum injuries

clear correlation between the outcome and initial MR finding in this series.

Only in one case was surgery indicated by the MRI finding alone, and this was a case of suboccipital acute epidural haematoma (Fig. 3).

Discussion

The CT scan is a tool sufficiently accurate for surgical decision making in acute head injury, as it has weakpoints in the skull base, posterior fossa and also in fine non-haemorrhagic lesions. Otherwise, MR is very device concerning central nervous system disorder, including head injury and is now being discussed. We shall be able to detect smaller fine lesions if more high-field tesla and examination times are possibble. However MRI had significantly better specificity and sensitivity than CT in central structure injuries.

It is natural to consider that the severity of the primary brain injury may be correlated with central structural damage. Attempts have been made to correlate CT findings with pathological reports of primary brain stem

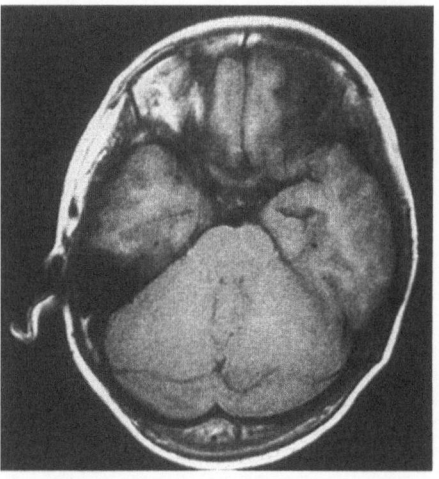

Fig. 3. 7 year-old. Posterior fossa acute epidural haematoma. The Haematoma shows iso-intensity and the dura shows linear low-intensity. T1 weighted image (SE, TR1000/TE 30). On CT, haematoma shows iso-density and might be missed

injury[7], for example DAI. However it must be recognized that DAI is an essentially purely pathological entity[5]. At present it is impossible to apply these imaging methods at the ultrastructural level for accurate neurobehavioural assesment[4]. Therefore we consciously avoided the use of such terms in describing MRI findings. MRI findings cannot and should no the used to evaluate injury at the cellular level. From the findings obtainable at present the only applicable term to be used for the CT or MR findings of such lesions is such as tissue tear haemorrhag[6].

Brain injuries involve extremely complex factors and there are also many MRI parameters. While CT scan is at present more advantageous for acute head injuries because of its speed if MR could be performed in a shorter period of time it would replace the CT procedure.

References

1. Adams JH, Graham DI, Murray LS, *et al* (1982) Diffuse axonal injury due to nonmissile head injury is humans. Ann Neurol 12: 557–563

2. Kelly AB, Zimmerman RD, Snow RB, Gandy SE, Heier LA, Deck MDF (1988) Head trauma: comparison of MR and CT-experience in 100 Patients. AJNR 9: 699–708
3. Gentry LR, Thompson B, Godersky JC (1988) Trauma to the corpus callosum: MR Features. AJNR 9: 1129–1138
4. Levin HS, Amparo E, Eisenberg HM, *et al* (1987) Magnetic resonance imaging and computerized tomography in relation to the neurobehavioral sequelae of mild and moderate head injuries. J Neurosurg 66: 706–713
5. Strich SJ (1956) Diffuse degeneration of the cerebral white matter in severe dementia following head injury. J Neurol Neurosurg Psychiatry 19: 163–185
6. Willberger JE Jr, Rothfus WE, Tabas J, Goldberg AL, Deeb Z (1990) Acute tissue tear hemorrhage of the brain: computed tomography and clinicopathological correlations. Neurosurgery 27: 208–213
7. Zimmerman RA, Bialnuik LA, Genneralli T (1978) Computed tomography of shearing injuries of the white matter. Radiology 127: 393–396

Correspondence: Dr. T. Ogawa, Department of Neurosurgery, St. Marianna University School of Medicine, Yokohama City Seibu Hospital, 1197-1 Yasashi-cho, Asahi-Ku, Yokohama 241, Japan.

Acta Neurochir (1992) [Suppl] 55: 11–13

HM-PAO Spect in Head Trauma

J.M. Gonçalves[1], **R. Vaz**[1], **A. Cerejo**[1], **C. Cruz**[1], **J. Pereira**[2], **A. Mourão**[2], and **I. Amaral**[2]

[1] Neurology and Neurosurgery Department, Hospital de S. João, Porto, Portugal, [2] Nuclear Medicine and Biophysics Department, Faculty of Medicine, Porto, Portugal

Summary

Single Photon Emission Computed Tomography (SPECT) after intravenous administration of Technetium-99m hexamethylpropylene-amine oxime (Tc-99m HM-PAO) makes possible the evaluation of cerebral perfusion.

We have been assesssing the diagnostic accuracy of SPECT in some groups of head trauma patients: the preliminary results of this study are presented.

Fourteen patients have been selected, all of them showing some kind of focal neurological deficit; the Computed Tomography (CT) and Nuclear Magnetic Resonance (NMR) were normal, or showed lesions that could not be responsible for the neurological deficits. In all of the patients Tc-99m HM-PAO SPECT has been performed, showing changes in cerebral perfusion in areas correlated with the abnormalities elicited on clinical examination.

These results show that Tc-99m HM-PAO SPECT is a better technique than CT or NMR in demonstrating the organic basis of some neurological deficits observed after head trauma.

Keywords: Head trauma; HM-PAO SPECT; brain blood perfusion; radionuclide studies.

Introduction

Single Photon Emission Computed Tomography (SPECT) after intravenous administration of TC-99m labelled hexamethypropylene-amine oxime (HM-PAO) has been used in the evaluation of the brain blood perfusion in several clinical settings: stroke, epilepsy, dementias and brain tumours are examples[2, 3, 4, 5, 6, 7, 8]. In neurotraumatology, however, its use has been quite limited, but it has been demonstrated that Tc-99m HM-PAO SPECT can show more lesions and at an earlier stage than CT[1]. This is not surprising since the technique has not only the capability of showing anatomical lesions but also functional abnormalities, namely brain blood perfusion asymetries.

In head trauma we are ocasionally faced with patients presenting with focal neurological deficits but with a CT and NMR normal or showing lesions not directly related with the observed deficits.

The aim of our work was to investigate if, in this group of patients, there were brain blood perfusion abnormalities and, if so, that they could be correlated with the observed deficits.

Materials and Methods

Fourteen patients with the above mentioned conditions have been selected. Eleven were admited in our neurotraumatology unit after road traffic accidents and three after a fall. Table 1 shows our series. Twelve patients were aged below fourty five years. The Glasgow Coma Score (GCS) was equal or greater than thirteen in twelve patients and the neurological deficit was hemiparesis in eleven patients. There were no other neurological abnormalities and the past medical history, taken either from the patient or their relatives, was irrelevant.

All these patients underwent a CT scan on the same day of the Tc- 99m HM-PAO (SPECT). Since NMR is not available in our hospital it was not possible to perform this study on the same day, but the delay was not greater than one week.

NMR was not performed in two patients who had metallic prosthesis because of associated bone trauma.

All the patients underwent a SPECT starting 10 to 15 minutes after intravenous administration of 25 mCi (925 MBeq) of Tc-99m HM-PAO. This compound not only quickly crosses the blood brain barrier and distributes itself in the cortex proportionally to the blood perfusion but also remains there long enough to allow the acquisition of data for the tomographic reconstruction.

Sixty-four 40s frames were collected on a 64×64 matrix using a general purpose collimator fitted to a General Electric Maxi-Camera/400T interfaced to a Gamma 11 System. Reconstruction of data was made by filtered back projection of profiles (SPECT) using the softest filter and no attenuation correction. Transverse sagittal and coronal sections with 13 mm nominal tickness were obtained.

In all cases it was possible to obtain scans of good quality which were evaluated by a nuclear medicine physician who did not know the findings the neurological examination nor the CT or NMR images.

Table 1. *Clinical Characteristics of Patients*

	Name	Age	GCS	Neurological deficits
1	AMFS	18	15	right hemiparesis (+ face and arm)
2	EJM	19		aphasia
3	ARSB	60	10	aphasia; focal seizures
4	MHCL	23	10	aphasia
5	ARS	47	15	right hemiparesis
6	FJSR	19	13	right hemiparesis (+ face and arm)
7	VMLS	17	15	left hemiparesis
8	JMOL	28	14	right hemiparesis
9	ASP	41	15	left hemiparesis
10	MFS	21	15	left hemiparesis
11	AMT	25	13	right hemiparesis
12	JMR	32	14	right hemiparesis (+ face and arm)
13	AMRG	41	15	left hemiparesis
14	MAST	22	14	right hemiparesis

+ = Prevailing.

Results

The CT and NMR were normal in all patients except in case 2 presenting with bilateral frontal hygromas and cases 4 and 11 with some degree of brain atrophy. The NMR was not obtained in patient 11 for the above mentioned reasons.

The Tc-99m HM-PAO SPECT results are shown in Table 2. None of the patients had a normal brain blood perfusion: we found a clear relationship between the neurological deficits and the distribution of the abnormalities on the brain blood perfusions.

Discussion

This work shows that Tc-99m HM-PAO SPECT is able to show functional abnormalities triggered by head trauma, even when the CT scans and NMR images are normal.

The decreased perfusions can be the result of altered regional cerebral blood flow regulation as a direct consequence of head trauma, or a secondary phenomenon of metabolic abnormalities. In any case these alterations are not severe enough to cause anatomical changes that could be seen on CT or NMR.

Its prognostic capabilities and possible therapeutic implications are yet to be established.

Table 2. *TC-99m HM-PAO SPECT Results*

	Name	Neurological deficits	SPECT
1	AMFS	right hemiparesis (+ face and arm)	decreased perfusion (left parieto-temporal)
2	EJM	aphasia	decreased perfusion (left parieto-temporal)
3	ARSB	aphasia; focal seizures	right/left asymmetry
4	MHCL	aphasia	decreased perfusion (left temporo-temporal)
5	ARS	right hemiparesis	decreased perfusion (left parietal) small focal perfusion deficit (left frontal)
6	FJSR	right hemiparesis (+ face and arm)	decreased perfusion (left fronto-parieto-temporal)
7	VMLS	left hemiparesis	decreased perfusion (right parietal) small focal perfusion deficit (right temporal)
8	JMOL	right hemiparesis	decreased perfusion (left fronto-parieto-temporal)
9	ASP	left hemiparesis	decreased perfusion (right parieto-temporal)
10	MFS	left hemiparesis	decreased perfusion (right fronto-parietal)
11	AMT	right hemiparesis	decreased perfusion (left fronto-parietal)
12	JMR	right hemiparesis (+ face and arm)	decreased perfusion (left parietal)
13	AMRG	left hemiparesis	decreased perfusion (right parieto-temporal)
14	MAST	right hemiparesis	decreased perfusion (left parietal)

+ = Prevailing.

In some selected cases Tc-99m HM-PAO SPECT can be a powerful ancillary test able to give us some insight into the complex pathophysiological events triggered by head trauma.

References

1. Abdel-Dayem HM, Sadek SA, Kouris, *et al* (1987) Changes in cerebral perfusion after acute head injury: comparison of CT with Tc-99m HM-PAO SPECT. Radiology 165 (1): 221–226
2. Andersen AR, Gram L, Kjaer L, *et al* (1987) SPECT in parcial epilepsy: identifying side of focus. Acta Neurol Scand [Suppl 78] 117: 90–94

3. Dressler D, Voth E, Feldmann M, *et al* (1989) The development of an epileptogenic focus. A case study with 99m Tc-HM-PAO SPECT. J Neurol 236 (5): 300–302

4. Goldenberg G, Podreka I, Suess E (1989) The cerebral localization of neuropsychological impairment in Alzheimer's disease: a SPECT study. J Neurol 263 (3): 131–138

5. Langen KJ, Roosen N, Herzog H, *et al* (1989) Investigation of brain tumors with 99Tcm HMPAO SPECT. Nucl Med Commun 10 (5): 325–334

6. Leys D, Steinling M, Petit H, *et al* (1989) Maladie d'Alzheimer: étude par tomographie d'émission monophotonique (HMPAO Tc [99m]). Rev Neurol 145 (6–7): 443–450

7. Smith FW, Donald RT, Morris AJ, *et al* (1988) The study of regional cerebral blood flow in stroke patients with technetium 99m HMPAO. Br J Radiol 61 (275): 358–361

8. Yeh SH, Lin RS, Hu HH, *et al* (1986) Brain SPECT imaging with 99Tcm-hexamethylpropyleneamine oxime in the early detection of cerebral infraction: comparison with transmission computed tomography. Nucl Med Commun 7 (12): 873-878

Correspondence: JM Gonçalves, MSc, MD, Departments of Neurology and Neurosurgery, Hospital de S. João, 4100 Porto (Portugal).

Acta Neurochir (1992) [Suppl] 55: 14–17

Early Post-Traumatic Cerebral Blood Flow Mapping: Correlation with Structural Damage After Focal Injury

R. Bullock[1], **D. Sakas**[1], **J. Patterson**[2], **D. Wyper**[2], **D. Hadley**[3], **W. Maxwell**[4], and **G. M. Teasdale**[1]

[1] Department of Neurosurgery, University of Glasgow, [2] Department of Clinical Physics, [3] Department of Neuroradiology,
[4] Institute of Neurological Sciences, Glasgow, Department of Anatomy, University of Glasgow, Glasgow

Summary

Focal post traumatic mass lesions such as contusions and intracerebral haematomas are common, and often difficult for neurosurgeons to manage, because little is known of their pathophysiology. We have mapped cerebral blood flow, and studied small vessel ultrastructure at different time points within the first three weeks of head injury, in patients with these lesions.

A zone of ischaemic brain is always present around these lesions, and persists for weeks or months. This accords with astrocyte swelling and microvascular compression seen on electron microscopy.

Focal zones of hyperaemia were also present in 42% of patients, within the first two weeks of injury, and this appeared only within apparently normal tissue as judged by late MRI or CT.

Keywords: Contusion; cerebral blood flow; brain ischaemia; electron microscopy.

Introduction

Mass lesions are the commonest cause of preventable death after head injury, and they are also frequently responsible for long-term neuropsychological deficit in survivors[8,13,14]. In a few patients, cerebral contusions may swell and enlarge to cause worsening brain shift, raised intracranial pressure and even death, yet the mechanisms by which these changes occur are not fully understood[3,6]. Although the histology of cerebral contusions has been well described, the most striking feature is the neuronal and astrocytic degeneration and pyknosis which extends for many millimetres or even centimetres beyond the limits of the haemorrhagic lesion, which is the hallmark of a contusion[10]. Although Lindenberg and Freytag speculated in 1957 that a shear mechanism maybe responsible for this extensive zone of pyknotic change around a contusion, there have been few published studies directed at this problem[4,6,8,10]. In order to improve understanding of the pathophysiological mechanisms causing brain demage after a cerebral contusion, we have related regional cerebral blood flow changes early after focal head injury to the changes seen on structural imaging such as CT and MRI. To correlate these CBF changes with microvascular anatomical abnormalities, we have also performed ultrastructural studies of the tissue at the edge of a focal cerebral contusion in 18 patients who underwent surgery for removal of large mass lesions.

Patients and Methods

We have performed regional cerebral blood flow mapping studies using 99mTc HMPAO (1200 mbq) in 43 patients with CT demonstrated focal lesions. The first scan was performed within 21 days of injury in all these patients. SPECT studies were performed using a NOVO 810 head dedicated imager. Twenty-one of these patients were studied on more than one occasion, 24 hours to three months apart. In seven patients with acute subdural haematomas, and five patients with acute extradurals, blood flow studies were obtained with the haematomas in situ. For these studies, the first pass binding characteristics of HMPAO were utilised as follows[1]. HMPAO was injected as soon as the haematoma was diagnosed by CT scan, and before taking the patient to theatre for craniotomy and haematoma evacuation. Immediately after haematoma evacuation, the patient was imaged using the SPECT scanner. HMPAO reamins bound to cerebral tissue for about five to six hours in proportion to blood flow passing through the brain at the time of injection, so that images which represent the blood flow distribution with the haematoma in situ may be obtained after the haematoma has been removed[1,7].

The SPECT images were correlated with CT or MRI scans performed within 48 hours of the SPECT study. Because of uncertainties regarding the mathematical modelling of HMPAO uptake and back diffusion from brain, cerebral blood flow could not be calculated from the tomographic images[1]. Analysis of SPECT images was performed by measuring regional HMPAO uptake and comparing this with HMPAO uptake, in medial occipital cortex, a region which we found to be unaffected after head injury, in our experience of over 120 post-traumatic scans.

Regional hyperaemia was recorded when HMPAO uptake was greater than that seen in the medial occipital cortex. Clinical features in the patients studied were recorded onto data collection forms, and compared with changes on SPECT and structural imaging.

Ultrastructural Studies[4]

In a different group of 18 patients who underwent surgical removal of a focal cerebral contusion, biopsies were taken from the margins of the contusion bed after removal of the necrotic contusion tissue. Biopsy specimens were immediately immersion fixed in Karnoffsky's fixative. Specimens were taken from three hours to twenty days after injury. These were compared to control specimens taken and fixed in the same way, from normal tissue in patients undergoing temporal lobectomy for epilepsy or tumour. After processing for electron microscopy, a minimum of 10 vascular regions from each biopsy were studied and particular attention was paid to vascular and perivascular ultrastructure, studied both by transmission and scanning electronmicroscopy.

Results

Focal Cerebral Contusion

In every patient with a significant cerebral contusion or intracerebral haematoma (> approximately 1.5 cms diameter) a zone of reduced cerebral blood flow was present around the lesion (Fig. 1). Such ischaemic zones were usually larger than the haemorrhagic lesion itself but not greater than the extent of the T_2 weighted MRI lesion corresponding to the surrounding oedema. Partial volume considerations limit the conclusions which can be drawn about the size of the ischaemic areas (resolution of the SPECT imager = ± 0.8 cm). In most of the patients who underwent serial imaging, the ischaemic zone became smaller with time: in two patients the ischaemic zone appeared larger when SPECT scanning was performed three months after injury.

Hyperaemic Zones (Tables 1 and 2)

Hyperaemia was seen in 18 of 43 patients (42%) but it was only seen on scans performed within 14 days of injury with the exception of a single case in which hyperaemia persisted on a second scan three weeks after injury. The zones of hyperaemia appeared to affect both white and grey matter and were directly adjacent to ischaemic zones. Hyperaemia was never seen within the contusion itself, or within tissue which on MRI appeared to have high "T_2 weighted" signal intensity, indicating oedema.

Hyperaemia, therefore, always appeared to occur within normal tissue as judged by CT or MRI. Nine patients in whom hyperaemia had been present were serially scanned, and the hyperaemia had dissappeared by

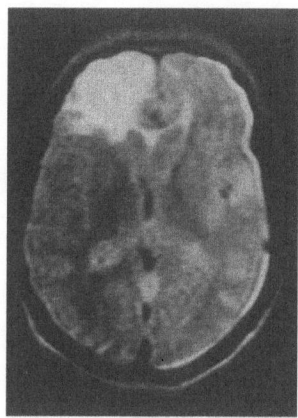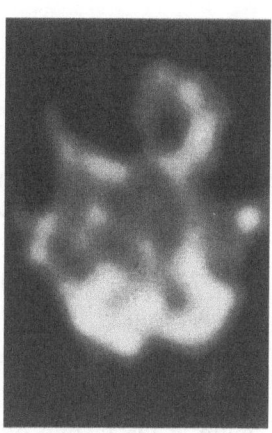

Fig. 1. Left frontal contusion. Left: "T_2 weighted" MRI scan. Note large zone of high signal intensity related to the left frontal contusion and ill-defined zone of high signal intensity in the right temporal region. Right: HMPAO SPECT mapping study. Note the zone of profoundly reduced CBF in relation to the left frontal and right temporal contusions

Table 1. *Relationship of Hyperaemia to Structural Brain Lesions*

	Hyperaemia	No hyperaemia
Contusion	10	9
Intracerebral haematoma	5	7
Sbdural haematoma	1	6
Extradural haematoma	2	3
	18	25

Table 2. *Relationship of Hyperaemia to Outcome at 3 Months*

Outcome	Good result	Maximally disabled	Severely disabled	Dead
Hyperaemia	14	9	2	1
No hyperaemia	10	8	3	2
	31		8	

the third week in all but one patient. When late CT or MRI was performed in this group of patients, the previously hyperaemic tissue appeared to be structurally normal on imaging.

Clinical Features and Outcome in Patients with Hyperaemia

Hemiparesis was present in four patients with hyperaemia, and in three without. The mean age of these hyperaemic patients was 53 years. The incidence of skull fracture was similar in patients with and without hyperaemia as was the incidence of coma on admission. Outcome was slightly better in patients with hyperaemia than in those without when tested at three months using the Glasgow Outcome Scale (Table 2).

CBF Mapping with Acute Subdural and Extradural Haematoma

Hyperaemia was seen in two of the five patients with acute extradural haematomas, in one it was present ab initio at the margin of the zone of tissue which was compressed by the extradural haematoma (Fig. 2).

In the second patient, hyperaemia developed 24 hours after the extradural haematoma was removed, most marked in the contralateral frontal region. A zone of reduced CBF was seen immediatly underlying the extradural haematoma in all five patients, but this was mild even when the extradural haematoma was large. Hyperaemia was present in only one of the seven patients with acute subdural haematomas, and in this patient a small contusion was also present underlying the subdural. In two of the patients with acute subdural haematomas a marked and extensive zone of blood flow reduction was present under the subdural, but in the other two no change in CBF pattern could be detected.

Ultrastructural Changes

The most significant feature on transmission electronmicroscopy was massive swelling of astrocytes. Astrocyte perivascular foot process swelling was particularly marked and this was maximal at 24 to 48 hours after injury, regressing markedly by five days. In many specimens, astrocytic foot process swelling was suffi-

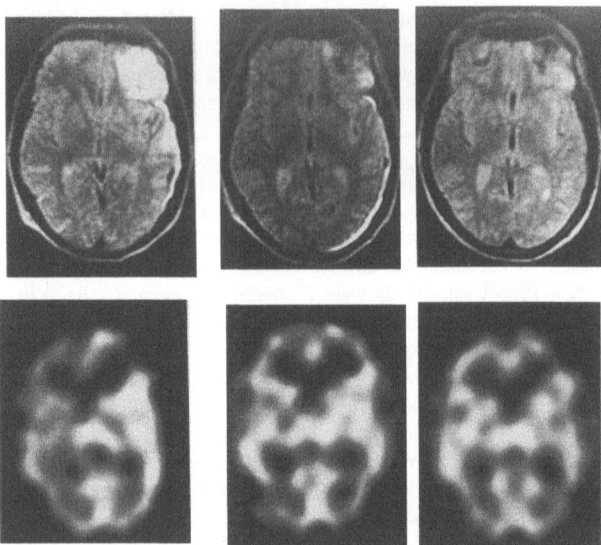

Fig. 3. Right hemisphere hyperaemic zone in relation to a small right frontal contusion and very thin "smear" subdural haematoma over the right hemisphere. Top row: "T_2 weighted" MRI scans performed at five (left) 15 (middle) and 40 days after head injury (right). Bottom row: Matching SPECT CBF maps. Note the zone of hyperaemia in the right parieto-temporal and frontal regions which has disappeared by 15 days

cient to cause compression and even occlusion of the lumen of some capillaries. No gross changes were seen in the morphology of capillary endothelial cells, but micro-vacuole formation was depressed. Tight interendothelial junctions were intact in all specimens studied. Neuronal morphology appeared to be relatively better preserved in specimens taken within the first few hours after injury and was most abnormal in specimens taken more than 12 hours post injury.

MRI Imaging

In all patients with focal contusions or intracerebral haematomas, large zones of high signal intensity were seen on T_2 weighted scans suggesting marked cerebral oedema in relation to these focal lesions. No consistent MRI pattern was noted in relation to hyperaemia (Figs. 1 and 3).

Discussion

There is no clear consensus in the neurosurgical literature regarding the optimal management of patients with focal post-traumatic lesions who remain in a stable neurological condition[3, 7, 8]. This is because the pathophysiology of both focal contusion and intracerebral

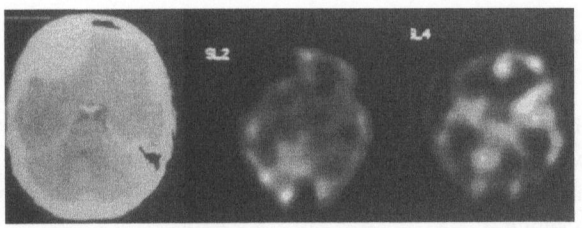

Fig. 2. Acute extradural haematoma imaged 16 hours after injury. Left: CT scan. Centre: SPECT HMPAO image. HMPAO injected at the same time as CT scan on left, but image obtained after haematoma has been removed. Right: HMPAO CBF map obtained five days after haematoma removal. Note zone of mild hyperaemia in the contralateral frontal region

haematoma remains poorly understood. In particular, there is little understanding regarding the mechanisms by which these lesions cause damage to surrounding brain tissue.

The three major findings in these studies are:

1. All significant (> 1.5 cm) traumatic intraparenchymal lesions induce a zone of severely reduced CBF in the surrounding brain. This zone of reduced CBF persists for days, weeks or even months in many cases.

2. Massive astrocyte swelling may cause capillary compression early after the injury, and be the cause of the reduced focal CBF.

There is no evidence for 'vasospasm' in the periphery of these lesions[4].

3. Focal hyperaemia is a frequent (42%) and apparently benign, transient phenomenon persisting up to two weeks after focal injury, which takes place chiefly in *normal* tissue, adjacent to intraparenchymal or extracerebral lesion.

The first of two of these findings accord closely with results from animal models of intracerebral haematoma[2, 5, 11].

The focal hyperaemia seen in these patients differs from the patterns reported in animal models, in which hyperaemia seems to be global and much shorter, persisting for minutes or hours, only depending on the severity of the antecedent ischaemic insult[9]. Our studies, however did not include patients with severe diffuse head injury, as did those of Obrist *et al.*[12].

The implications of these studies for clinicians who care for neurotrauma patients are several. Drugs which enhance CBF would be unlikely to improve focal perilesional perfusion. However, drugs which are capable of limiting astrocyte swelling, may be of value when given early. These may include aminosteroids, other free radical scavengers, calcium antagonists, and glutamate antagonists (see page 49, this volume).

Contusions and intracerebral haematomas are always surrounded by a zone of ischaemic tissue and pyknotic, dead neurons, so that those exerting mass effect should be resected when necessary to control ICP, in the knowledge that viable tissue will not be jeopardised.

References

1. Anderson AR (1989) 99mTcD, 1-hexamethylene-propylene amine oxime (99mTc HMPAO): basic kinetic studies of a tracer of cerebral blood flow. Cerebrovasc Brain Metab Rev 1: 288–318

2. Bullock R, Brock-Utne J, van Dellen JR, Blake G (1988) Intracerebral haemorrhage in a primate model: effects on regional cerebral blood flow. Surg Neurol 29: 101–107
3. Bullock R, Golek J, Blake G (1989) Traumatic intracranial haematoma: which patients should undergo surgical evacuation? CT scan features and ICP monitoring as a basis for decision making. Surg Neurol 32: 181–187
4. Bullock R, Maxwell WL, Graham DI, Teasdale GM, Adams JH (1990) Glial swelling following human cerebral contusion: an ultrastructural study. J Neurol Neurosurg Psychiatry (in press)
5. Bullock R, Mendelow AD, Teasdale GM, Graham DI (1982) Intracranial haemorrhage induced at arterial pressure in the rat. I. Description of technique, ICP changes and neuropathological findings. Neurol Res 6: 184–188
6. Bullock R, Statham P, Patterson J, Teasdale GM (1990) Vasogenic oedema after focal human head injury – a SPECT mapping study. In: Reulen HJ, Baethmann A, Marmarou A (eds) Brain Edema VIII. Proceedings of the Eight International Symposium, Berne, June 17–20, 1990. Acta Neurochir (Wien) [Suppl] 51: 286–288
7. Bullock R, Statham P, Patterson J, Teasdale GM, Teasdale E, Wyper D (1989) Tomographic mapping of CBF, CBV and blood brain barrier changes in humans after focal head injury using SPECT: mechanisms for late deterioration. In: Hoff J, Beks JL (eds) Intracranial pressure VII. Proceedings of the 7th International Symposium, Ann Arbor, June 19–23, 1988. Springer, Berlin Heidelberg New York, pp 637–640
8. Bullock R, Teasdale GM (1990) Head injuries – surgical management: traumatic intracranial haematomas. Chapter 10. In: Baakman R (ed) Vinken and Bruyn's Handbook of Clinical Neurology, Vol 13 (57). Head injury. Elsevier Science Publishers, Amsterdam, pp 249–296
9. Ginsberg MD, Budd WW, Welsh FA (1978) Diffuse cerebral ischaemia in the cat. I. Local cerebral blood flow suring ischaemia and recirculation. Ann Neurol 3: 482–492
10. Lindenberg R, Freytag E (1957) Morphology of cortical contusions. Arch Pathol 63: 23–42
11. Mendelow AD, Bullock R, Teasdale GM, Graham DI, McCulloch J (1984) Intracranial haemorrhage induced at arterial pressure in the rat. II. Short term changes in local cerebral blood flow measured by autoradiography. Neurol Res 6: 189–194
12. Obrist WD, Langfitt TW, Jaggi JL (1984) Cerebral blood flow and metabolism in comatose patients with acute head injury. Relationship to intracranial hypertension. J Neurosurg 61: 241–253
13. Reilly PL, Adams JH, Graham DI, Jennett B (1975) Patients with head injury who talk and die. Lancet 2: 375–377
14. Wiedmann KD, Patterson J, Hadley DM, Bullock R (1988) Correlates of focal lesions in closed head injury: distribution of cerebral blood flow and neuropsychological performance. J Clin Exp Neuropsychol 11: 1–58

Correspondence: Dr. R. Bullock, University Department of Neurosurgery, Institute of Neurological Sciences, Southern General Hospital, Glasgow G51 4TF, U.K.

Acta Neurochir (1992) [Suppl] 55: 18–20

The Role of Computer Based Techniques in Patient Monitoring: Technical Note

P. Guedes de Oliveira[1], **J. P. Cunha**[1], and **A. Martins da Silva**[2]

[1] INESC/University of Aveiro, [2] Serviço Neurofisiologia, Hospital Geral de Santo António, Porto, Portugal

Summary

In this paper the requirements of Neurophysiology and Neuro-traumatology monitoring are analyzed. As a result a set of designated systems were developed by the authors a short description of which is given in the paper. Finally the future perspectives and problems to be faced are briefly described.

Keywords: Monitoring; EEG; computer based system multimedia; archiving.

The Problems Raised by Monitoring

The problems we have to face in monitoring in neuro-traumatology and, in general, in neurophysiology reside essentially in two facts: first, the long duration of monitoring sessions – implying a large amount of data to analyze and store – and second the different nature of the data to be monitored simultaneously; in fact, we are concerned with an environment where we have various types of biological signals – EEG, ECG, respiratory variables, etc. – and, frequently, the video-image of the patient, if available, would conveny important information.

This diversity, raises some fundamental questions:

- how to store the large amount of data;
- how to synchronize the different types of information;
- how to retrieve the data, efficiently;
- how to process the data (in real-time or off-line);
- how to extract higher level information from the raw data.

All these aspects require technological, computer-based means that may become helpful tools to the physician both in diagnosis and prognosis as well as in helping him or her in deciding and acting as soon as the situation requires.

Our Approach to Facing some of These Questions

To face this complex environment we have been engaged in the development, application and testing of a set computer-based systems, different in their very essence but aiming at solving some of the problems as stated above:

– The first of these systems is HIDRA-Hierarchical Instrument for Distributed Real-Time Analysis[3] which is a multiprocessor system the hierarchical natural of which allows, at the lower level, the separate processing of various channels of data and, at a higher level, the integration of information in order to derive interchannel relationships. The independence of the low level processors makes it easy to install and debug processing software, adequate to each type of analysis to be performed. Another important feature of HIDRA is that it is a real-time system, processing the data as it comes, which may be a

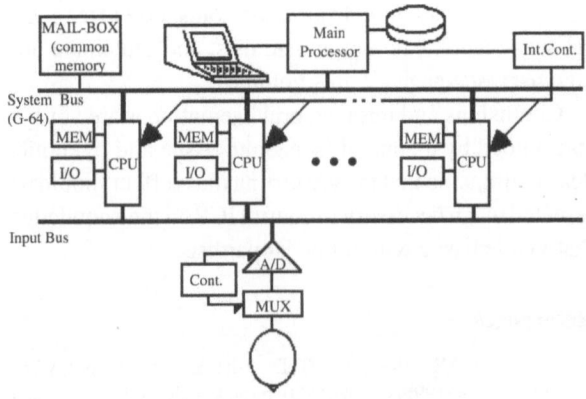

Fig. 1. Hidra is a tightly coupled multiprocessor system in which the various processors share 2 buses: the first one where they have access to a multiplexed digital version of the input signals and the 2nd one that gives access to a shared memory and which is also the main processor's bus

very important fact for, e.g., alarm generation. To achieve the real-time capabilities both for channel per channel and inter-channel analysis, HIDRA interprocessor coupling is tied through what is normally designated as a shared memory scheme. Finally, HIDRA has been used mainly in epilepsy and sleep studies but is as well adapted for e.g., coma monitoring.

– DORIS – Digital Overlaid Recording of Image and Signal[2] is another system which has proved to be very important in our monitoring routine. It aims at offering a possible solution to the problems of storage of large amounts of data, multimedia storage and, finally, synchronization. What the system really does is to record in a common medium (a Video Cassette) a high quality version of up to 16 channels of data (12 bits/sample, 800 samples/sec/channel), together with an analog black and white image. These two sets of information are totally independent, as far as the recording process is concerned, but are, nevertheless, intrinsically synchronized. This allows separate retrieval and processing of the data signals, its conversion to analog form (for paper recording, for instance) but also the inspection of the detailed image that corresponds to some specific event detected in the signals. For this purpose, the system generates a clock that is visible on the TV screen and also registered on tape, made available for paper output and also for computer analysis.

– Finally, we have been engaged in the development of KISS – Knowledge-based Interactive Signal monitoring System[1*]. KISS aims at integrating the real-time monitoring of signals with knowledge-based analysis and decision. The goal of the project is to develop a general framework for monitoring systems, based on this philosophy and to build and test a prototype applied to Coronary Care Units (CCU). The reason for choosing a CCU as the application environment has to do with the interest and experience of the clinical partterns in the consortium but the goal of a general monitoring framework makes KISS useful for other applications.

The Architecture of KISS has recovered the hierarchial nature developed and tested with HIDRA, and the prototype was built as two separate sub-systems (low- and high-level) communicating by a network link; the coupling is not as tight as it was in HIDRA and a standard Ethernet connection was chosen. For the low-level sub-system an AT compatible computer was chosen, running MS-DOS; it acquires the signals, converts them to digital and performs the signal analysis and pre-processing. From this analysis, features are extracted and events detected and passed to the high-level subsystem, which is a Unix based machine. For the communication the socket mechanism is used. At the high level an application dependent knowledge base is being built which is able to anlayze the features in order to derive higher level, more elaborate conclusions.

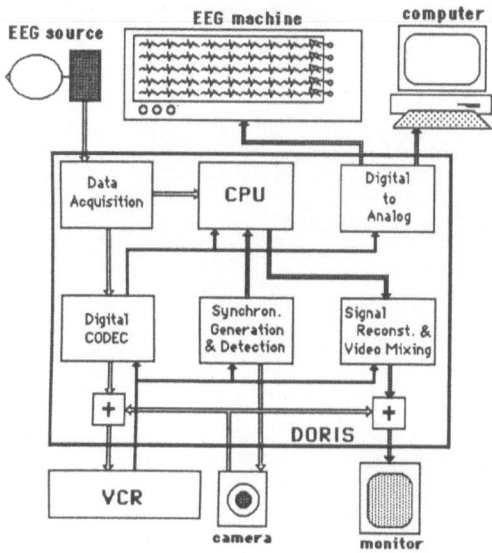

Fig. 2. DORIS is a recording system in which a VTR is used to record in a synchronized way both analog image and a digitalized version of 16 analog signals (normally EEG) sampled at 800 Hz per channel. The system allows an independent retrieval of image and signal and recreates the signal overlayed on the video screen

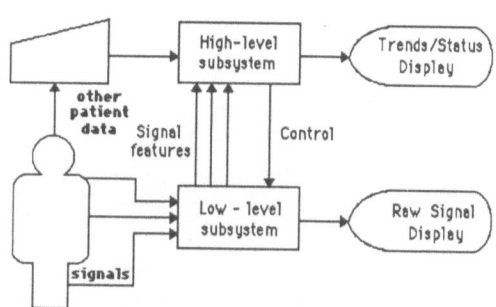

Fig. 3. In KISS the hierarchical processing concept was further developed to implement an intelligent, knowledge based interactive monitoring system: in our prototype low and high level sub-systems communicate through an Ethernet LAN

---

*KISS is a project supported by ECC program AIM of DG-XIII. The first author of this paper was responsible for the participation of INESC in this project. The other members of the consortium were VOLMAC (NL) who was the project leader, the University of Rennes I (F), the University of Bradford (UK), the Centro de Bioingigneria and the National Research Institute (I) and RACIA (F)

Future Perspectives

After a number of years of work in the neurophysiology monitoring field, our perspective is that the systems that we developed and described above are partial, non-integrated answers to some of the questions we iniatially asked. The main effort in the near future will therefore be in integration. This has to be approached at two levels:

– at the hardware level, by building a network which takes the information from the various systems and makes it available in a common medium and format;

– at the software level, i. e., at a level where the information that was gathered and analyzed with separate goals adds up, in order to increase the knowledge and the confidence, for advising the physician and help in his or her decision for further treatment. This is definitely the most challenging task which we will approach by means of IKBS's (Intelligent Knowledge Based Systems). In order to do that, we have started the process of building a neurophysiology knowledge-base, focusing on the three main topics of activity which have been pursued in our group: traumatology, epilepsy and sleep studies.

This task was the goal of a project submitted and approved by JNICT (the Portuguese Applied Science Agency) started in January 91.

References

1. Belshaw JC, Ferreira PJ, Garner VP, Guedes de Oliveira P, Oliveira e Silva T, Luz Vieira JH (1991) The KISS prototype: a validation platform for a knowledge-based real-time monitoring system. In: Proceedings of the 1st European Conference on Biomedical Engineering, pp 233–234
2. Cunha MB, Guedes de Oliveira P, Príncipe JC (1990) Integrated system for simultaneous recording and display of image and signal, SINFHOS 90 – Symposium Informática Hospitalária, Barcelona, 1990, cs 23
3. Guedes de Oliveira, P, Príncipe, JC, Cruz, A, Tomé, AM (1987) HIDRA – a hierarchical instrument for distributed real-time analysis of biological signals. In: IEEE Transactions on BME, pp 921–927

Correspondence: Prof. P. Guedes de Oliveira, Departamento Electrónica e Telecomunicações, INESC, Universidade de Aveiro, 3800 Aveiro, Portugal.

Acta Neurochir (1992) [Suppl] 55: 21–24

Significance of Endocrine Studies in the General Assessment and Prediction of Fatal Outcome in Head Injury

T. Pentelényi

National Institute of Traumatology, Department of Neurosurgery, Budapest, Hungary

Summary

Serial basal blood glucose, serum insulin, cortisol, growth hormone, glucagon and catecholamine examinations were performed in 81 brain-injured patients. 32 patients with severe injuries of other parts of the body (chest, abdomen, limbs or polytrauma), and 17 patients with non-traumatic acute brain lesions served as double control. In the brain-injured patients there is a close relation between changes of the state of consciousness and those of basal blood glucose levels: the deeper coma the higher and wider is the pathological glucose-level range. Four types of blood-glucose changes could be identified in the background of which different alterations of each hormone level were observed.

Fatal outcome could be predicted in a non-diabetic patient in the first days when seeing:

1) Fasting hyperglycaemia above 14 mmol/1; 2) Fluctuating basal blood glucose levels between 5 and 22 mmol/1; 3) Deeply depressed and unchanged basal insulin level; 4) Extremely high cortisol level; 5) Decreased plasma epinephrine level.

These changes in the carbohydrate metabolism seen after acute brain lesions are not identical to diabetes mellitus.

Keywords: Blood glucose; serum hormone levels; brain injury; state of consciousness; prognosis.

Introduction

What kind of endocrine changes of the carbohydrate metabolism are caused by severe acute traumatic brain lesions in a non-diabetic patient? Do any of these changes have prognostic significance? Do they need endocrine correction, and are they of the same nature as those in diabetes mellitus?

These were the basic questions which we aimed to answer in a long-range prospective clinical study.

Material and Methods

Serial laboratory tests were taken in 130 patients of the National Institute of Traumatology, Department of Neurosurgery and ICU during the course of five years. Daily examinations of basal blood glucose, serum insulin, cortisol, growth hormone, glucagon, nor-epinephrine and epinephrine levels were made in three groups of patients: 1) 81 brain-injured patients; 2) 32 patients with other injuries: chest, abdomen, limbs or polytrauma; 3) 17 patients with non-traumatic acute brain lesions: subarachnoid haemorrhage, apoplexy, tumours etc.

Venous fasting blood samples were taken daily till recovery or death during the first three weeks. To record the disturbance of consciousness the *Fischgold-Matis* coma-scale was used[1]. The neurological picture was followed daily, pathology identified by diagnostic procedures was proved in many cases by operation and/or autopsy.

Determination of blood glucose was performed by the ortho-toluidine method.

The insulin level was determined by measuring the quantity of serum immuno-reactive insulin (IRI). Double antibody method was used according to *Hales and Randle*. Examinations were made with Amersham kits[2].

Determinations of non-conjugated 11-hydroxycorticoid levels (cortisol and corticosterone) were performed by *Mattingly's* fluorimetric method[6].

In the serum growth hormone determination partly the CIS method was used - this is based on double antibody techniques - and partly the Phadebas HGH PRIST method in which paper-disc was applied as solid phase[14, 15].

The method of determination of plasma glucagon level was a radio-immunoassay (*Korányi et al.*) which was suitable for determining only the activity of pancreas glucagon without that of enteroglucagon[4, 5].

Determinations of plasma catecholamines - nor-epinephrine and epinephrine – were carried out by radio-enzymatic methods according to *Versteeg et al.*[16, 17].

Data were analysed and evaluated by computerised data processing, applied different statistical methods.

Results

1. There are well defined differences between the changes of the basal blood glucose level in brain-injured patients and patients with other severe injuries[8].

2. In the clinical neurological picture the *state of consciousness* seemed to be correlated with the *basal*

blood glucose level.. Coma caused by brain injury is accompanied by elevation of blood glucose, improvement of consciousness by normalisation of glucose level. There is a quantitative correlation between the severity of coma and the degree of hyperglycaemia: the deeper the coma the higher and wider is the blood glucose range[8, 12], Fig. 1.

3. In the background of the blood glucose changes simultanous alterations of the basal plasma hormone levels were found: very low insulin level, extremely high glucagon and cortisol levels, moderate elevation in the catecholamine levels, and after an initial high peak continuous low growth hormone level[11, 13].

4. According to the registered endocrine changes *four types* of brain-injured patients could be separated. Typical features of each type are mathematically verified and illustrated in Fig. 2, together with the actual changes in the state of consciousness[10].

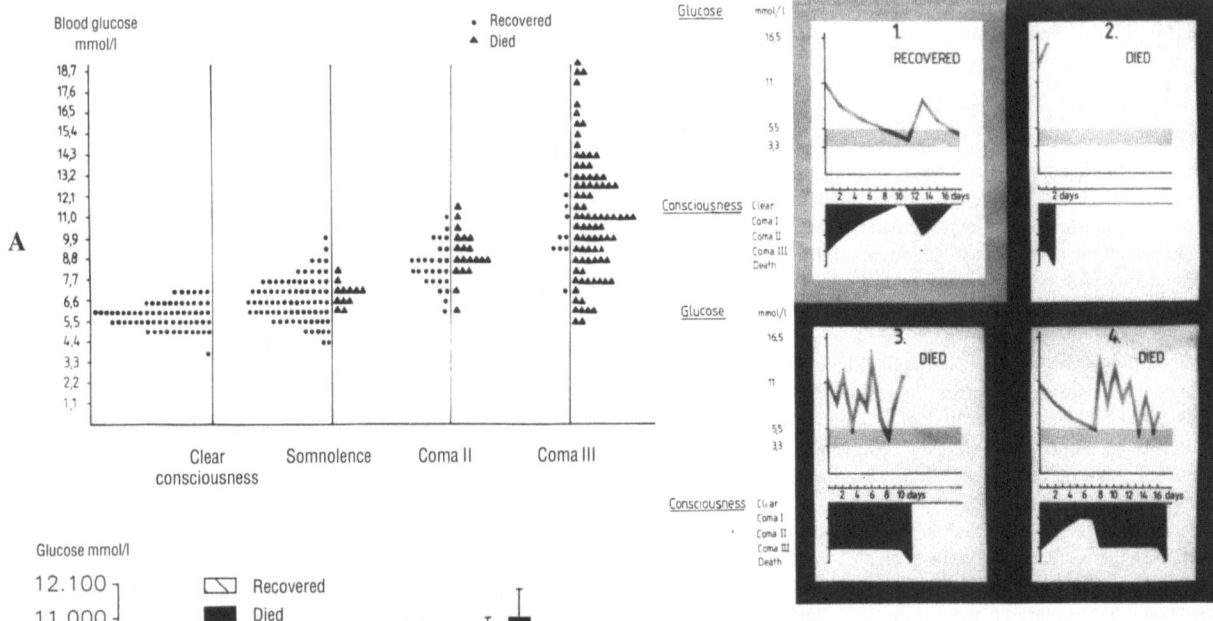

Fig. 2. Basal blood glucose changes in brain injured patients. New head injury classifying system based on endocrine changes which clarifies the relationships between hormonal changes, alterations in the state of consciousness and clinical course. Of the four charts the first relates to the patient who recovered, the other three to those who died. State of consciousness according to the Fischgold-Matis coma-scale.

In the *first type* an elevated fasting glucose level was found in comatose patients. Together with the improvement of the state of consciuosness normalisation of the glucose level was observed. If the patient got into deeper coma again, the blood glucose was elevated concurrently. If the conscious level improved glucose level was normalised again. The most seriously injured patients belonged to the *second type*: they died in 48 hours. Basal blood glucose was in most cases above 12 mmol/l. In the *third type* lethally injured patients were alive for 1-2 weeks. During this period big fluctuations of the glucose level were seen along with unchanged deep coma. In the patients of the *fourth type* there was a temporary improvement in the state of consciousness with a decrease of hyperglycaemia. But because of severe complication deep coma and rapid elevation of the glucose level was observed. In the next period permanent deep coma was seen with fluctuating and gradual decreasing of blood glucose levels

Fig. 1. (A) Individual values of basal blood glucose levels taken in the first 48 hours after brain injury in patients with different states of consciousness. (B) Statistical evaluation of the data above of the patient-groups with different states of conciousness. In both figures the Fischgold-Matis coma scale was used (data of 300 tests)

Similar characteristic changes were identified in the different hormone levels mentioned above type by type, but there is no possibility to show them in such a short paper[10,13].

Discussion

Among the endocrine patholophysiological data there are some which do have prognostic significance. Fatal outcome can be predicted in the first days when finding any of the results below in a non-diabetic brain-injured patient[9, 10]:

1) Fasting hyperglycaemia above 14 mmol/1. Fig. 3[3, 7, 8].

2) Fluctuating basal blood glucose level between 5 and 22 mmol/1.

3) Deeply depressed and unchanged insulin level, against big fluctuations of the blood glucose level.

4) Extremely high cortisol level.

5) Decreased plasma epinephrine level.

Of course these endocrine changes are not the causes of the fatal outcome. They are severe katabolistic consequences of the same irreversible brain damage which causes both deep coma and death. According to the results of correlation and cross-correlation studies the deeper the coma the looser are the physiological endocrine correlations. In coma stage III complete endocrine dissociation can be observed which is most crucial in the carbohydrate metabolism of the whole organism[10].

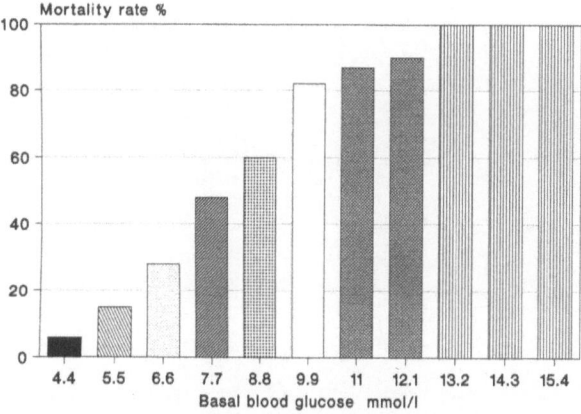

Fig. 3. Correlation between the mortality and the basal blood glucose level of the brain injured patients. The graph shows that the mortality rate of those patients whose basal blood glucose level ranged from 8.8–9.8 mmol/1 in the first 48 hours, was 60 per cent, etc. The critical basal blood glucose level of non-diabetic brain-injured patients was 13.2 mmol/1, above this level no survival was seen among 500 patients

The hyperglycaemia of severe brain-injured patients – most often 11–22 mmol/1 values – does not generally need endocrine treatment. Decreasing of the high blood glucose level by *insulin administration* in most cases is *unnecessary* and what is more it can be *dangerous*. It is unnecessary since there are only two conditions: the keto-acidotic state and hyperosmolaric coma in which insulin treatment is absolutely indicated but these conditions generally do not occur as consequences of brain injury in the early stage.

It is *dangerous* because lowering of the blood glucose level by insulin treatment diminishes plasma oncotic pressure, thus it can enhance the possibility of brain oedema and its most severe consequence:hippocampal herniation. On the other hand decreasing of the blood glucose level can cause further deterioration in the metabolism of the injured brain.

As a result of severe brain injury special changes ensue in the endocrine pancreatic function: in spite of hyperglycaemia the insulin level stays low and glucagon level becomes extremely high. This divergence of bicellular function seems to be of a *functional nature in brain-injured patients* in contrast with the *organic lesion of the islet system in diabetic patients*.

Although someone can find certain changes in brain-injured patients' endocrine constellation which can be similar either to those of the diabetes of the adult type (predominance of contra-insular hormones) or those of juvenile diabetes (relative lack of insulin), disturbances of carbohydrate metabolism caused by brain injury are not identical with diabetes mellitus.

There is no loss of capability for insulin secretion since glucose-loading is followed by a considerable "insulin-answer". It is the central regulation of the pancreatic endocrine function which is damaged, and as a consequence of it the "functional rigidity" of the beta and alpha cells develops by a marked decrease of glucose-sensitivity[7, 10].

Conclusions

1. Changes in the blood glucose and different hormone levels caused by brain injury are specific for brain injury if compared with those of patients with other injuries, but they do not differ in their essentials from the alterations of patients with non-traumatic brain lesions (of course with the exception of hypothalamic local pathology).

2. Among the examinations of prognostic value the basal blood glucose test is the most simple and in-

formative one. It is worth while to take into consideration its significance during the first days after head injury regarding the prediction of the late outcome.

References

1. Fischgold H, Matis P (1959) Obnubilations, comas et stupeurs. Masson et Cie, Paris
2. Hales CN, Randle PJ (1963) Immunoassay of insulin with insulin-antibody precipitate. Biochemistry J 88: 137
3. Keymolen-Jardini V, Mouawad E, Claeys de Clercq P, *et al* (1974) Glucose Matabolism in Traumatic Brain Injury. Acta Endocrinol 77: 103
4. Korányi L, Péterfy F, Paksy A, Vargha P (1977) Production of glucagon antibodies by Thyroglobulin-Zinc glucagon conjugate. Horm Metab Res 9: 434
5. Korányi L, Péterfy F, Tulassay Zs, Papp J, Pentelényi T, Tamás Gy JR (1977) Methodological problems of radioimmunological glucagon determination. Diabetol Croatica 5: 43
6. Mattingly D (1962) A simple fluorimetric method for the estimation of free 11-hydrocorticoids in human plasma. J Clin Path 15: 374
7. Mouawad E, van Laere E (1974) Traumatisme cranien et diabete sucre attitude therapeutique. Ann Anesth Franc 15: 355
8. Pentelényi T, Kammerer L (1977) Changes in blood glucose after head injury. Injury 8: 264
9. Pentelényi T, Kammerer L (1977) Blood glucose reflects outcome in head injury. Medical Monitor 2: 9–14
10. Pentelényi T (1978) Effect of brain injury on the fasting blood glucose and hormone levels characterising carbohydrate metabolism. Thesis of C.Sc., Hungarian Academy of Sciences, Budapest
11. Pentelényi T, Kammerer L, Stützel M, Balázsi I (1979) Alterations of the basal serum insulin and blood glucose in brain-injured patients. Injury 10: 201
12. Pentelényi T, Bezegh A, Fekete M, Kammerer L, Korányi L, Péter F, Stützel M, Veress G (1981) Endocrine changes caused by acute traumatic and non-traumatic brain lesions. Neurological Surgery. Thieme, Stuttgart New York. Neurochirurgia (Stuttg) [Suppl]: 188
13. Pentelényi T, Kammerer L (1984) Alterations of the serum cortisol and blood glucose in brain-injured patients. Injury 15: 397
14. Schalch DS, Parker ML (1964) A sensitive double antibody immunoassay for human growth hormone in plasma. Nature: 203, 1141
15. Thorell J (1976) Phadebas HGH PRIST. Clinical and technical information. Pharmacia Diagnostics AB. Almquist and Wiksell, Uppsala
16. Versteeg DHG, Van der Gugten J, Van Ree JM (1975) Regional turnover and synthesis of catecholamines in rat hypothalamus. Nature: 256, 502
17. Versteeg DHG, Palkovits M, Ven der Gugten J, Wijnen HLJM, Smeets GWM, de Jong W (1976) Catecholamine content of individual brain regions of spontaneously hypertensive rats(SH-rats). Bain Res 112:429

Correspondence: Dr. T. Pentelényi, National Institute of Traumatology, Department of Neurosurgery, Budapest, Hungary.

Acta Neurochir (1992) [Suppl] 55: 25–28

Blunt Basal Head Trauma: Aspects of Unconsciousness

K. Boström[1], **C.-G. Helander**[1], and **S. Lindgren**[2]

Departments of [1] Forensic Medicine and [2] Neurosurgery, University of Göteborg, Göteborg, Sweden

Summary

Two cases of street violence directed to the skull base level and transverse to the cervical axis are described. No skeletal damage. The violence resulted in the so-called "traumatic subarachnoid haemorrhage", an often used, unspecified forensic "diagnosis"; it was here revealed to be due to rupture of the wall of the posterior inferior cerebellar artery (p.i.c.a).

However, this was only one of the possible explanations for the acute symptoms of unconsciousness (concussion) and almost immediate death.

The careful examination of these two cases and of a series of control cases revealed that at the trauma, stress and strain may have occurred to arterial branches serving as feeding perforant vessels to the medulla oblongata; in these cases they were coursing directly from the p.i.c.a. region. – The type of direct impact has often been regarded as mild! However, its location suboccipitally as in these cases can become dangerous.

The resulting direct or indirect deficit of brain stem functions are discussed in these cases as well as "concussion-related symptoms" resulting after other types of head and neck injury.

Keywords: Head trauma; unconsciousness; concussion; cerebral dysfunction; brain stem.

Introduction

It is well known that closed head injuries may be described with different clinical pictures and courses in cases observed clinically, cases examined by hospital-pathologists or described in forensic material. This is due to the different severity of the primary damage, complications occurring but also to different types of injury.

We will describe forensic cases after street violence where injury and haemorrhage of the posterior inferior cerebellar artery (p.i.c.a.) have occurred with very short survival. Considering the "mild" character of the trauma, the site of impact and the related local anatomy may be of great significance. The simultaneous traumatic unconsciousness is discussed and also compared with "concussion" and other posttraumatic symptoms related to other types of head and neck trauma.

Case Reports

The first case was a 29 year old man assaulted by fists and kicks to his body and finally a karate blow to his neck suboccipitally. He immediately became unconscious and arrived at the hospital with respiratory arrest and cardiac arrest. At autopsy a 4 × 2 cm fresh haemorrhage was found in the neck muscles, in the midline reaching the skull base at the foramen magnum. Extensive subarachnoid haemorrhage was found with the cisterns filled with blood and blood in the ventricles. There were no cortical contusions. At microscopical examination the brainstem was of normal appearance. Half a centimeter peripheral to the origin of the p.i.c.a. from the vertebral artery there was a 2 mm rupture in the vessel wall. Close to the rupture a small branch left the p.i.c.a. to the medulla.

The next case was a 24 year old man assaulted by two men with two fist blows to the right side of his face. He almost fainted and sat down on a bench. After another fist blow to the right side of his face from the other man he immediately became unconscious and was dead at the arrival to the hospital. At the autopsy small bruises were found on the right side of the nose, in the right zygomatic region and in the upper and lower lip. To the right of the transverse process of the atlas a 2 × 2 cm haemorrhage extensive subarachnoid drainage in the cisterns and the ventricles. There were no cortical contusions. At microscopical examination the brain stem appeared normal.

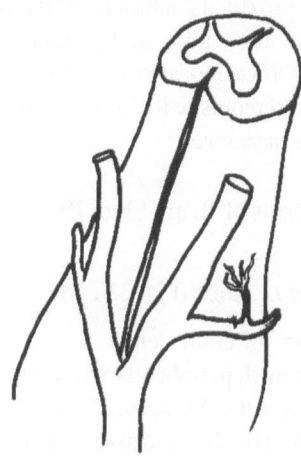

Fig. 1. Site of rupture of posterior inferior cerebellar artery (p.i.c.a.) related to the branch to medulla oblongata

The right p.i.c.a. showed a 2 mm rupture on its ventral aspect 1 cm after branching off from the vertebral artery. Immediately distal to the rupture a small arterial perforator coursed directly into the medulla oblongata.

Discussion

The occurrence of the pathophysiological denominator "Coma" has been related to terms of global physical Head Injury Criteria (HIC) or Head Injury Coma Criterion (HICC) based on acceleration and time. The *local* anatomical characteristics can also be of importance, particularly at the cranio-spinal junction including the skull base and brain stem.

The p.i.c.a. has a highly varying anatomical course and some branches may leave it directly for the medulla or have a circumflex course around part of the lateral and anterior surface of the medulla (Fig. 1).

1. ANATOMICAL PREREQUISITE

PICA FIXED TO MEDULA OBLONGATA

2. TRANSVERSE HORIZONTAL IMPACT
|
STRAIN OF PICA
|
RUPTURE OF PICA

Fig. 2. Probable local anatomical and biomechanical prerequisites for injury of intracranial p.i.c.a.

In a consecutive autopsy-material of 43 cases with 143 branches from the proximal centimeter of the p.i.c.a. we found only 4 branches with a direct course into the medulla. This was revealed also in the two cases described, forming a prerequisite for injury of specific local trauma at the skull base level.

Possible Mechanisms of Brain Stem Dysfunction
(Fig. 3)

Tissue Mechanical Damage (Fig. 3A, B)

A. "Concussion" of brain stem.

B. The small branch peripheral to the arterial rupture and fixed to the medulla oblongata, with a peripherally directed strain was possibly a cause of impairment of brain stem functions such as unconsciousness and respiratory arrest.

A.

CONCUSSION OF BRAIN STEM
|
BRAIN STEM DYSFUNCTION

B.

ANCHORING ARTERY
|
INDIRECT STRAIN ON MEDULLA
|
BRAIN STEM DYSFUNCTION

C.

"FEEDING" ARTERY

RUPTURE   LOCAL
HAEMORRHAGE   VASOSPASM

ISCHAEMIA

BRAIN STEM DYSFUNCTION

D.

SUBARACHNOID HAEMORRHAGE
|
RAISED INTRACRANIAL PRESSURE
|
ISCHAEMIA
|
BRAIN STEM DYSFUNCTION

Fig. 3. Possible mechanisms of brain stem dysfunction at trauma to the skull base level

Vascular Damage (Fig. 3 B, C)

Strain might develop in that part of the vessel proximal to the rupture site and probably be the cause of the rupture.

C. The perforator anchored to the medulla oblongata was also a feeding artery and the strain could cause vasospasm or rupture, producing brain stem ischaemia and dysfunction.

D. The clinical course seemed similar to many fatal subarachnoid haemorrhages from ruptured arterial aneurysms.

Krauland[4] described the so called forensic diagnosis

"Traumatic subarachnoid haemorrhage" occurring mostly after fights or falls with impact to face or occiput and often unconsciousness or death immediately or within minutes. He reviewed 27 published cases and four new observations; it was assumed, without further anatomical analysis, that in 16 cases of lacerations of arteries from the circle of Willis overstretching might be a factor in these ruptures. In eight cases there were longitudinal ruptures free from branches, so called bursting ruptures and in the four new cases the 4–5 mm long ruptures were situated near branching of the p.i.c.a. Usually only bruises and abrasions in the face were observed and sometimes fractures of the skull and mandible but only once injury to the cervical vertebrae.

The relative rarity of published cases such as those described can be due to the rarity of the observation of special anatomical factors required in spite of the often occurring street violence.

The courses of the described cases may also fit the concept used some decades ago of *"experimental animal brain concussion"* with resulting serious disturbance of respiration and cardiovascular function together with the occurrence of coma (and absence of corneal reflexes).

This could indicate *"brain stem concussion"*.

Experiments were described[1] to differentiate the cervicospinal angular movement from the whiplash movements with mobile skull by fixating the skull of rhesus monkeys and impacting the body in a forward direction. The result was instantaneous alterations in blood pressure, heart rate, respiratory rate, spinal cord conduction and a concussion-like state; they did not observe what they called "experimental concussion unless cervical spinal cord injury" was produced.

In this respect the results were similar to those of so called "percussion concussion".

In a review[3] of "cranial nerve palsies in cervical injuries" in eight patients a man was reported hit by a falling tree resulting in a fractured spinous process C4 (but no other skeletal damage). He became unconscious, and on regaining consciousness he was found to have a spastic tetraparesis and bulbar palsy. He also had a soft tissue swelling around the ligamentum nuchae. He recovered within 8 weeks.

It is also well known that patients with cervical cord injury from angular movement or penetrating injuries can show mental dysfunction and confusion-syndromes.

There are many case reports of hyper-extension-flexion "whiplash" *amnesia and confusion* occurring in car passengers (in seat belts) and observed awake or transiently unconscious (s.c. "concussion") when the car has been struck from behind. The memory disturbances have been referred to *"hippocampal-fornical system"*[2] injuries.

In a consecutive series over 2 years 2600 head injuries[8] were reported with various groups of assumed "brain stem lesions" in 240 cases. In only one fourth, 60 patients, the clinical course suggested primary brain stem lesions and they appeared to have damage at the bulbar or pontine level. The bulbar cases died while the pontine (6 cases) "could have" preservation of other brain stem and higher cerebral functions. In a case of "locked in syndrome"[7] on MR-scanning a large sharply demarcated lesion (infarction) was found in the pons in a 36-year old woman; it appeared after cervical manipulation and she was mutistic but awake and tetraplegic, probably due to external compression-stretching or vasospasm of the vertebral artery.

The clinical concept *"human cerebral concussion"* includes posttraumatically impaired general attention, confusion syndromes "disorganisation and incoherence of thoughts and speech" and different types of amnesia.

In severe head trauma the various clinical pictures mentioned may be added to each other. – A more basic difficulty in defining coma or unconsciousness in the particular patient is that part of the "consciousness" complex is damaged: the process generator of arousal-wakefulness, of awareness-cognition or of memory (amnesia)-emotional-autonomic structures.

Clinical diagnoses can not possibly grade severity levels of the condition of the particular case when based only on general neuropathological knowledge. However, this has been used particularly by English and American authors for example "diffuse axonal injuries", or "diffuse shearing axonal injuries". It is not possible to know the mechanics in the particular case, but morphological alterations may be revealed by MR, if available. "Multiple focal injuries" seem sometimes a more appropriate morphological description. The classification has been mixed up with clinical terms! These differences have caused many difficulties in terminology as well as in understanding of the mechanisms involved in posttraumatic impairment of consciousness.

For semantic clarity Ommaya[6] in a "consensus workshop" recommended the use of the diagnoses of the clinical conditions observed (cf. Lindgren[5]) commonly done by European investigators.

The presented two cases indicate that other kinetics and biomechanics in direct craniospinal injuries may cause other pathophysiological changes in "closed head injury" than those usually discussed in human head injuries.

References

1. Coe JE, Calvin TH, Rudenberg FH, Yew CH (1967) Concussion-like state following cervical cord injury in the monkey. J Trauma 7: 512–522
2. Fisher CM (1982) Whiplash amnesia. Neurology NY 32: 667–668
3. Grundy DJ, McSweeney T, Francis Jones HW (1984) Cranial nerve palsies in cervical injuries. Spine 9: 339–343
4. Krauland (1981) Die traumatische subarachnoidale Blutung. Z Rechtsmed 87: 1–18
5. Lindgren S (1986)Diagnostic terminology of head injuries-related to severity. In: Lindgren S (ed) Modern concepts in neurotraumatology. Acta Neurochir (Wien) [Suppl] 36: 5, 70–80
6. Ommaya AK (1983) Physiopathology and biomechanics of head injury: introduction; diffuse injuries. In: Ommaya AK (ed) Head and neck injury criteria. A consensus workshop, NHTSA – USA, pp 19–20
7. Povlsen UJ, Kjaer L, Arlien S, Borg P (1987) Locked-in syndrome following cervical manipulation. Acta Neurol Scand 76: 486–488
8. Turazzi S, Alexandre A, Bricolo (1975) Incidence and significance of clinical signs of brain stem traumatic lesions. Study of 2600 head injured patients. J Neurol Sci 19: 215–222

Correspondence: Prof. Dr. S. Lindgren, Department of Neurosurgery, University of Göteborg, S-41345 Goteborg, Sweden.

Acta Neurochir (1992) [Suppl] 55: 29–32

Primary Traumatic Benign Midbrain Haematoma in Hyperextension Injuries of the Head

E. P. Sganzerla, P. M. Rampini, A. De Santis, F. Tiberio, P. Guerra, M. Zavanone, and G. Miserocchi

Institute of Neurosurgery, University of Milano, Milano, Italy

Summary

Primary traumatic brain stem injury occuring in isolation is not universally recognized as a distinct pathological entity which may follow a head injury. We describe two patients with clinical and radiological evidence of primary posttraumatic midbrain haemorrhage occuring in isolation associated with good recoveries. It is suggested that paramedian midbrain syndromes associated with midbrain haemorrhages should be recognized as a distinct, although unusual, complication of hyperextension injury to the head which may have a benign course.

Keywords: Head trauma; paramedian midbrain syndrome; midbrain haemorrhage; hyperxtension injury.

Introduction

It is usually stated that primary brainstem damage after head trauma is virtually always associated with widespread diffuse axonal injury or multiple petechial haemorrhages scattered throughout the brain[1, 2, 6, 15, 19].

Pontomedullary rent or separation[6, 7, 10, 14] and superficial contusions along the posterolateral aspect of the midbrain due to contact with the free edge of the tentorium[6, 8, 17] are considered the only possible exceptions.

Patients moreover with clinical evidence of brain stem damage after head injury rarely do well and are nearly always comatose from the initial impact[16].

In this report we describe two patients who, though fully conscious after head trauma, presented clinical and radiological evidence of focal midbrain damage with good recovery.

We suggest that paramedian midbrain syndromes associated with deep midbrain haemorrhages should be clinically recognized as a distinct, though unusual, type of primary traumatic brain stem damage which may occur in isolation and have a benign course.

Case Reports

Case 1:

M.G.M., a 30 years old male was admitted to the Department of Neurosurgery of the University of Milano on Dec 1, 1985. Two hours before admission, while driving his own car he was frontally struck by another car. In the emergency department vital signs were normal. Although drowsy, the patient could respond to verbal stimuli and follow complex commands. He was unable to open his right eye and the right pupil was dilated and fixed. Slight weakness of left limbs was also noted. Skull, cervical spine and chest X-rays were normal. CT scan showed a small focal haemorrhage placed in the upper part of the brainstem (Fig. 1). No supratentorial lesions could be detected. During the following days left motor weakness improved and drowsiness waned. On the 3rd day the patient was able to stand and eat unaided. Right 3rd nerve palsy was still

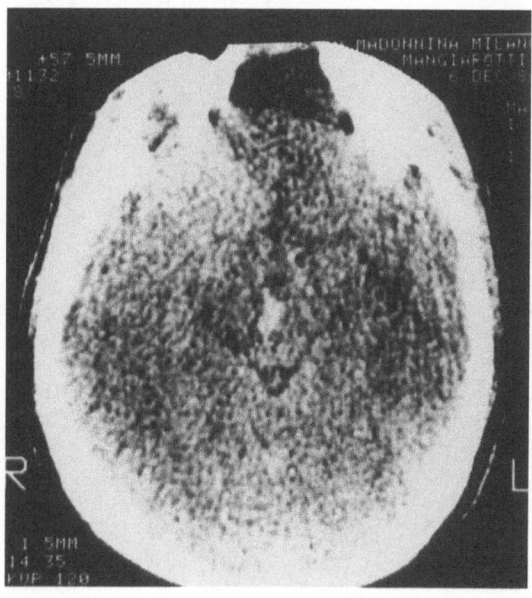

Fig. 1. Noncontrast-enhanced CT scan demonstrates a hyperdense lesion in the upper brain stem on the right side

complete and upward gaze paresis was present. High accuracy scans were repeated and showed the exact location of the midbrain haemorrhage and the absence of any other supratentorial or orbital lesion.

On follow-up examination one year later the patient, who meanwhile resumed his previous work, still presented a 3rd nerve palsy but had regained a normal pupil reactivity.

Case 2:

E. M. a 28 years old female was admitted the 18.9.89 following a road traffic accident in which her car was struck in the rear. On admission she was fully conscious and suffered from neck pain and diplopia. Ptosis of her right eyelid, anisocoria and diplopia on left conjugate eye movements together with slight weakness of her left arm were noted. Plain x-ray examination of her skull showed no fracture while cervical plain x-ray revealed a tear-drop fracture of C_2 (Fig. 2).

Computed tomography of the head showed a small area of high density in the midline of the upper brain stem (Fig. 3).

Magnetic resonance of the head showed a similar hyperintense lesion in the postero-inferior portion of the midbrain (Fig. 4).

Hospital stay was uneventful and on discharge strength of left arm was normal and oculomotor palsy was improving. At follow-up examination her neurological status was normal.

Discussion

Unilateral tegmental midbrain haemorrhages have been recognized as highly characteristic primary brain stem lesions by Crompton[4]. They were indeed the most

frequent finding in a series of 106 necropsies of patients dying soon after acute head injuries and occured in midbrains of normal, undistorted cross-sections.

A preponderance of occipital impacts was found in these patients, suggesting craniocervical displacements in a sagittal plane as an important pathogenetic factor in unilateral midbrain damage and assumed that primary haematomas could be the main cause of coma and short survival after head injuries.

Laum[9] describes primary brain stem haemorrhages caused by rhexis and observes that their site of predilection is, with decreasing frequency, the midbrain lateral sulcus opposite to the tentorial margin, the tegmentum and ventrally the irrigation area of intercrural branches of the basilar artery.

Mitchell and Adams[12] on the other hand, discussing pathological observations on 18 brain stems selected from a series of 100 fatal blunt head injuries, concluded that primary brain stem injuries do not exist as a pathological entity in isolation but are only an aspect of diffuse brain damage (diffuse axonal injury).

Occasional reports nevertheless indicate primary brainstem damage without lesions of the supratentorial region as a possible clinico-pathological event.

Shakir and Khan[18] describe a patient with internuclear

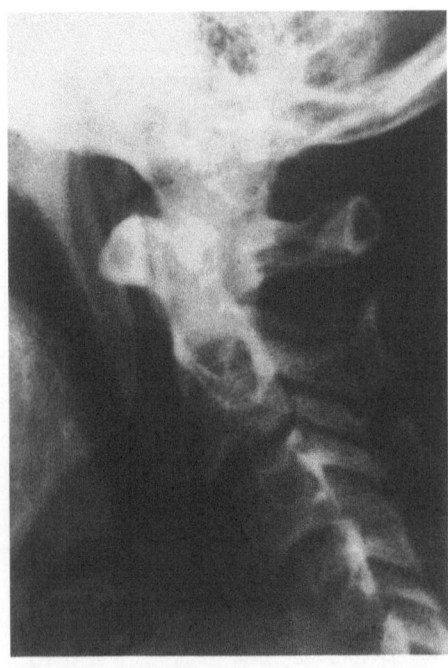

Fig. 2. Plain cervical x-ray shows a tear-drop fracture of C_2

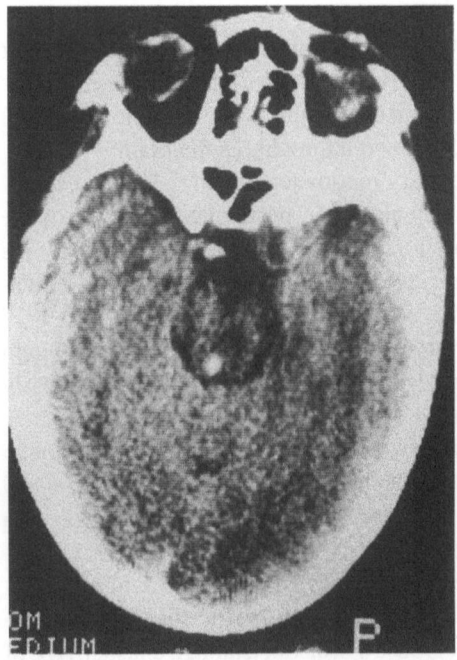

Fig. 3. CT scan without contrast agent shows a hyperdense lesion in the brainstem on the right

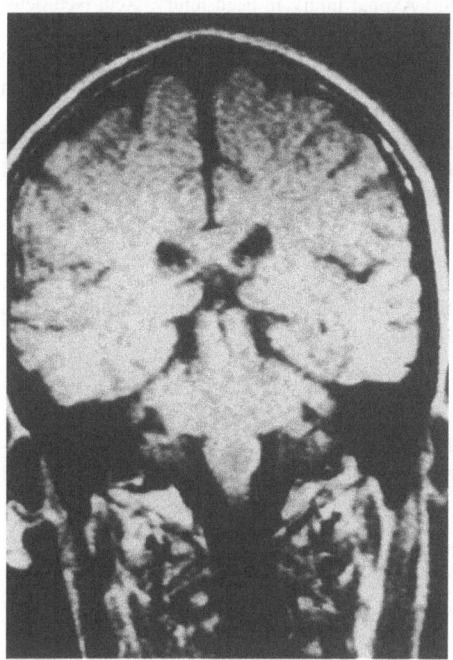

Fig. 4. Frontal MRI section of the brainstem shows a hyperintense lesion of the midbrain tegmentum

opthalmoplegia and truncal ataxia without impairment of consciousness after a head injury whose CT evidenced a small haematoma in the midline of the upper brain stem. The patient did well with complete resolution of neurological disturbances and resorption of the midbrain haematoma.

Davis[5] observes a similar case in which midbrain oedema suggesting a primary midbrain injury was associated with oculomotor disturbances and bilateral extensor posturing followed by recovery.

Pattisapu *et al.*[13] finally report an unilateral paramedian post-traumatic midbrain haemorrhage accompanied by preserved consciousness, decreased lateral gaze movements and skew deviation with bilateral extensor posturing to painful stimuli. This patient died following severe deterioration of his pulmonary status and septicaemia. Midbrain sectioning evidenced unilateral ovoid shaped haemorrhagic lesion of the left midbrain tegmentum occuring in an otherwise undistorted brain stem.

In both patients reported by us the CT located site of midbrain haemorrhage bears striking similarities with Crompton's and Laum's pathological specimens and definite clinico-radiological analogies with occasionaly reported clinical observations.

The affinity of all these cases and the almost constant presence of oculomotor palsies would indicate the me-

dian/paramedian midbrain as an area particularly vulnerable in head injuries.

In both our patients preservation of consciousness together with the absence of any clinical and/or radiological signs of supratentorial brain damage ruled out the possibility of diffuse damage to the white matter or of increased intracranial pressure with secondary brain stem damage.

C_2 anterior body fracture of Case 2 proved that impact produced severe craniocervical displacement in a sagittal plane with hyperextension of the head. Postero-anterior dislocation of the head as an important pathogenic factor in the production of focal traumatic midbrain damage has already been recognized by Crompton[4]. Bearing in mind the vascular supply of the midbrain and the similarity of clinical presentations to paramedian midbrain syndromes[3, 11] due to infarction in the territory of deep interpeduncular arteries, local vascular disruption due to stretching and tearing of deep perforating inter-peduncular arteries by tensile strains exerted along the anterior vascular structures during acute hyperextension trauma can be surmised.

Shearing may result from differential motility of brain stem and vessels, with basilar and vertebral arteries lagging behind in relation to the brain stem during acute anterosposterior displacements of the head.

We would suggest that paramedian midbrain syndromes associated with deep midbrain haemorrhage should be recognized as a distinct clinicopathological entity and considered as an existing, although unusual, primary brain stem damage which may occur in isolation and be associated with good recovery.

References

1. Adams JH, Graham DI, Scott G, Parker LS, Doyle D (1980) Brain damage in fatal non missile head injury. J Clin Pathol 33: 1132–1145
2. Adams JH, Gennarelli TA, Graham DI (1982) Brain damage in non missile head injury: observation in man and subhuman primates. In: Smith WT *et al* (eds) Recent advances in neuropathology, n 2. Churchill Livingstone, Edinburgh, pp 165–90
3. Claude H (1912) Syndrome pédonculaire de la region du noyau rouge. Rev Neurol 23: 311–313
4. Crompton (1971) Brainstem lesions due to closed head injury. Lancet i: 669–673
5. Davis RA (1983) Traumatic decerebrate rigidity and neurological recovery: a case report. Neurosurgery 12: 569–571
6. Gentry LR, Godersky JC, Thompson BH (1989) Traumatic brain stem injury: MR imaging. Radiology 171: 177–187
7. Harding B, Erdohazi M (1981) Traumatic transection of the brainstem. J Neurol Neurosurg Psychiatry 444: 1156–1158
8. Jellinger K, Seitelberger F (1970) Protracted posttraumatic encephalopathy: pathology, pathogenesis and clinical implications. J Neurol Sci 10: 51–94

9. Laum A (1990) Acute direct and indirect lesions of the brainstem. CT findings and their clinical evaluation. In: Primary and secondary brainstem lesions. Csécsei G, *et al* (eds) Primary and secondary brainstem lesions. Acta Neurochir (Wien) [Suppl] 40: 29–56

10. Lindberg R, Freytag E (1970) Brainstem lesions characteristic of traumatic hyperextension of the head. Arch Pathol 90: 509–515

11. Marie P, Guillain G (1938) Lésion ancienne du noyau rouge: dégénérations secondaires. Nouv Iconog Salpetriere 16: 71–74

12. Mitchell DE, Adams JH (1973) Primary focal impact damage to the brainstem in blunt head injuries. Does it exist? Lancet ii: 215–218

13. Pattisapu J, Smith RR, Bebin J (1985) Traumatic decerebracy with preserved consciouseness and voluntary movement. Neurosurgery 16: 71–74

14. Pilz P, Strohecker J, Grobovscek M (1982) Survival after traumatic ponto-medullary tear. J Neuro Neurosurg Psychiatry 45: 422–427

15. Pilz, P (1983) Axonal injury in head injury. Acta Neurochir (Wien) 32: 119–123

16. Rosenblum WI, Greenberg RP, Seelig JM, Becker DP (1981) Midbrain lesions: frequent and signicant prognostic feature in closed head injury. Neurosurgery 9: 613–620

17. Saeki N, Ito C, Ishige N, Oka N (1985) Traumatic brainstem contusion due to direct injury by tentorium cerebelli. Neurol Med Chir (Tokio) 25: 939–944

18. Shakir RA, Khan RA (1984) Traumatic brainstem haematoma without prolonged loss of consciousness. Brit Med J 288: 446–447

19. Tomlinson BE (1970) Brainstem lesions after head injury. J Clin Pathol 4: 154–165

Correspondence: Dr. Erik P. Sganzerla, Instituto di Neurochirurgia, Università Milano, via Francesco Sforza, 35, 20122 Milano, Italy.

Acta Neurochir (1992) [Suppl] 55: 33–36
© Springer-Verlag 1992

The Prognostic Value of some Clinical and Diagnostic Factors in Traumatic Intracranial Haematoma

A. Rudnik, M. Wojtacha, T. Wencel, and **P. Bazowski**

Neurosurgical Clinic, Silesian School of Medicine, Katowice, Poland

Summary

In order to carry out the analysis of predictive values of some clinical and diagnostic features, 146 patients of the Neurosurgical Clinic of the Silesian School of Medicine, were examined in 1980-1986. All the patients were in coma when admitted while CT findings showed traumatic intracranial haematomas. The examination included neurological diagnosis and CT examination. The analysis of statistical discrimination let us specify the probability of predicting death or survival of every patient. On the basis of 10 prognostic factors applied, the compatibility of prognosis and the real outcome for patients who survived was 78,2% and for those who died 91,2%.

Keywords: Head injury; prognosis; coma; computerized tomography; Glasgow Coma Scale.

Introduction

Traumatic intracranial haematomas constitute one of the more serious consequences of head injuries as they endanger the life of the patient and they are the cause of an uncertain and difficult prognosis. From the clinical point of view the designation of significant prognostic features in patients with traumatic intracranial haematomas allows to undertake, diagnostic and therapeutic procedures, commensurate with the gravity of the clinical state.

The recognition and standarization of values of separate prognostic features enables one to compare the results of procedures in various neurosurgical centers[3]. A new approach to the problem of prognosis for patients with severe head injuries has been presented in papers from the neurosurgical clinics in Richmond and Rotterdam[3,4,7]. Authors from these centers have used statistical-mathematical computer analysis of data for making a prognosis. Narayan[3] has used a linear logistical model of regression, a statistical program which takes advantage of a single datum or combination of data to obtain the final program for a single patient. The goal of the method used by Van Dongen[7], the so-called multinominal indenpen-dence model, was to choose a collection of the smallest number of features, which would contain the greatest number of available prognostic information.

Statistical discrimination analysis, used in this presentation, is a computer program which makes it possible to evaluate separate prognostic features, to establish a prognosis for each patient separately and to compare the results of prognosis with the actual state of affairs.

The aim of this paper was:

1) the evaluation of prognostic values of chosen features of clinical and CT examination in patients with traumatic intracranial injuries in cerebral coma,

2) the usage and evaluation of statistical discrimination analysis in making a prognosis for patients with traumatic intracranial haematoma in cerebral coma.

Materials and Methods

146 patients admitted to the Silesian Neurosurgical Clinic with severe head injuries between 1986–1989 were the subjects of this examination. The division of patients according to age is presented in Table 1.

Table 1. *Distribution of Age on Admission*

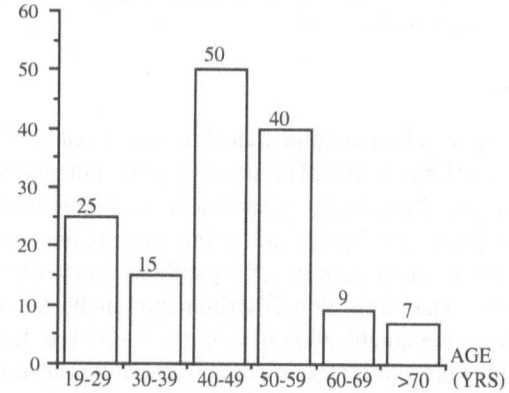

Table 2. *Patients Evolution in Function of the Ten Different Prognostic Factors*

Prognostic factor	1	2	3
I. Age	< 39 years	> 39 years	
II. GCS	6–8	3–5	
III. Motor response	correct	incorrect	
IV. Pupillary reaction	reacting	non reacting	
V. Vegetative disturbances	absent	present	
VI. Type of haematoma	epidural, subdural subacute and chronic haematoma	intracerebral and subdural acute haematoma	
VII. CT	subdural, epidural haematoma	subdural, epidural haematoma with single contusion or isolated intracerebral haematoma	subdural, epidural haematoma with multiple contusions or intracerebral haematoma with at least contusion focus
VIII. Shift of III ventricle	below 10 mm	above 10 mm	
IX. Widening of temporal horn on the opposite side to the haematoma	absent	present	
X. State of the basal cisterns	normal	partial obliteration	complete obliteration

1) Marked favourable changes; 2) less favourable changes; 3) unfavourable changes.

On admission all patients were in coma, ranging between 3 and 8 points on the Glasgow Coma Scale.

Based on CT findings, the presence of traumatic intracranial haematoma was established in all patients.

All but three, were operated upon. Statistical discrimination analysis was performed with the help of a series of mathematical-statistic analysis programs on a microcomputer.

In order to make a discrimination analysis, all patients were divided into two groups: those who survived and those who died. Ten examinations which had previously been evaluated from the point of view of their prognostic validity and statistical changeability were taken into consideration (Table 2).

It has been shown that some of these changes prognosed favourably and some unfavourably. Although the model of statistical discrimination is able to accept more than 2 input groups, in the majority of cases favourable prognostic changes were marked 1, and unfavourable – 2. Only in the case of the CT picture and the state of the basal cisterns, were the changes divided into three groups: marked favourable changes 1), less favourable changes 2), unfavourable prognostic changes 3).

Results

An analysis for a combination of features from I to V, i. e. age and four features of the neurological examination, the Glasgow Coma Scale appeared to be the factor of the greatest prognostic significance in this combination, followed by the motor response, the pupil reaction to light, age and vegetative reaction. Discrimination analysis conducted for the combination of features VI–X, i. e. five characteristics of CT examination showed that feature VII was the decisive one in this combination, followed by the state of the basal cisterns, the type of haematoma, the presence or absence of a widened temporal horn, and the degree of 3rd ventricle displacement.

Statistical discrimination analysis of all ten features showed that the Glasgow Scale of Coma has the greatest pronostic significance, the second being the degree of intracranial mass lesion which accompanies the haematoma.

The combination of prognostic features and the computer evaluation of their significance is presented in Table 3.

Table 3. *Prognostic Value of Clinical and CT Factors*

No.	Prognostic value
I	0.2472
II	0.7565
III	0.4714
IV	0.3906
V	0.0322
VI	0.2516
VII	0.6703
VIII	0.1282
IX	0.1382
X	0.4043

Table 4. *Relationship Between the Probability of Survival and Actual Outcome as a Function of Neurological, CT Examination or Both*

	Neurological examination		CT examination		NR + CT examination	
	I	II	I	II	I	II
Probability of survival	45	23	40	11	43	8
Probability of death	10	68	15	80	12	83
% of prognostic accuracy	81.8	74.7	72.7	87.9	78.2	91.2

I) Patients who actually survived; II) patients who actually died.

In this table the prognostic value is given in non-compound numbers which are the result of computer calculations. The value closer to 1,0 means a more prognostic value.

While making a discrimination analysis from the above 10 features the prognosis for survival and death for each patient were made separately. The probability of belonging to either a group which survived or died was calculated for each patient. The results were compared with the actual outcome. The dependence between the probability and actual outcome is presented in Table 4.

For the ten prognostic features the accuracy of prediction for the patients who survived was 78, 2% while for the ones who died it was 91,2%. For the five characteristics of the clinical examinations, it was respectively 81,8% and 74,7% and for five features of CT the accuracy of prediction it was 72,7% for patients who survived and 87,9% for the ones who died.

Discussion

Among the five clinical features, the Glasgow Coma Scale proved to be the strongest discriminator. In Narayan's findings, the Glasgow Scale also strongly prevailed over other clinical prognostic features. It should be remembered, however, that it is a complex examination. On the basis of computer discrimination analysis using five clinical features 81,8% of correct predictions of survival and 74,7% of correct predictions of death were established. The 25,3% of predictions which did not correspond to the actual state of affairs should be considered overoptimistic. It appears that errors of excessive optimism often result from complications which are not connected with the CNS trauma. Among them are: pneumonia, haemorrhage from the digestive tract, perforation of gastric ulcer, sepsis, circulatory and respiratory insufficency, orthopaedic injuries[7]. The tendency towards these complications increases with age. These non-neurological characteristics may significantly influence the course of treatment and the final prognosis. The difficulty in predicting complications of this kind can cause even the most perfect prognostic model to have flaws and become unreliable. However, as much as over-optimistic prognoses do not have unfavourable consequences for the patients, the consequences of to much pessimism may be more serious.

Ten patients (18,2%), for whom statistical analysis predicted death, and who actually survived, were under the influence of alcohol on admission to the hospital. It could have diminished reactiveness of patients and significantly lowered the clinical evaluation. Thus, this factor should also be stressed and given consideration, especially as it is often present in patients with head injuries.

The importance of a prognostic CT, both as a separate examination or as part of a set of other investigations has been given different value by different authors [1, 2, 3, 5, 6, 7].

Narayan[4] presents a rather sceptical view of its value as a separate examination, but adding it to a set of clinical factors increased the number of correct predictions in his opinion. Van Dongen[7], on the basis of a set or 4 tomographic features, in which the most significant feature was the state of the basal cisterns, showed a high prognostic value for the CT examination.

In this presentation, on the basis of 5 prognostic features, among which the most significant one was the degree of brain damage which accompanies the haematoma 72,7% of correct predictions of survival and 87, 9% of death were found.

It was shown that many patients with unfavourable changes in CT pictures survived. They constitute 27,2% of overoptimistic, erroneous predictions and prove the prognostic imperfections. In this case the errors in making a prognosis are perhaps due to a limited distributive ability of second generation tomographs, such as Somatom SD on which the examination for this work were performed. An erroneous prognosis for survival may also be due to the impossibility of finding small lesions of the brain stem, basal nuclei and parietal lobe.

The combing of prognostic features into one set consisting of ten variables increased the accuracy of prognosing death to 91,2%. The accuracy of predicting survival was 78,2% and did not surpass the accurancy of predictions on the basis of clinical features only, which was 81,8%. Using a large number of prognostic factors in the statistical analysis program increases the accuracy of making a prognosis, however not to the degree expected. Such a situation can be explained by the fact that various characteristics provide the same prognostic information.

To sum up, among the ten prognostic features considered in a discrimination analysis program the dominating role was assigned to the Glasgow Coma Scale and the state of the brain tissue in the CT picture. This program unabled an objective evaluation of prognostic features.

The determination of prognosis for a single patient on the basis of a combination of various clinical and tomographic features made it possible to prepare a combination which in future may be useful in predicting the fate of patients with traumatic intracranial haematoma.

References

1. Clifton GL, Grossman RG, Makela ME, *et al* (1980) Neurological course and correlated computerized tomography findings after severe closed head injury. J Neurosurg 52: 611–624
2. Heis E (1982) Die Prognose der akuten epiduralen Hämatome seit der Einführung der Computertomographie. Akt Traumatol 12: 1–3
3. Liesegang J, Siggelkow C, Weichert HC (1984) Computerotomografische in der Akutphase gedeckter Schädelhirnverletzungen. Neurochirurgia 27: 62–65
4. Narayan RK, Greenberg RP, Miller JD (1982) Improved confidence of outcome prediction in severe head injury. A comparative analysis of the clinical examination, multimodality evoked potentials, CT scanning and intracranial pressure. J Neurosurg 54: 751–752
5. Steiner J, Gomori JM, Melamed EM (1984) The prognostic value of the CT scan in conservatively treated patients with intracerebral haematoma. Stroke: 15, 2
6. Tsai FY, Huprich JE, Gardner FC (1978) Diagnostic and prognostic implications of computed tomography of head trauma. J Comput Assist Tomogr 2: 323–331
7. Van Dongen KJ, Braakman R, Gelpke GJ (1983) The prognostic value of computerized tomography in comatose head injured patients. J Neurosurg 59: 951–957

Correspondence: Dr. A. Rudnik, Neurosurgical Clinic, Silesian School of Medicine, Katowice, Poland.

Acta Neurochir (1992) [Suppl] 55: 37–39

Coexisting Diffuse Axonal Injury (DAI) and Outcome of Severe Head Injury

M. Shigemori, N. Kikuchi, T. Tokutomi, S. Ochiai, and **S. Kuramoto**

Department of Neurosurgery, Kurume University School of Medicine, Kurume, Japan

Summary

The importance of coexisting diffuse axonal injury (DAI) and outcome were studied in 107 patients with diffuse and focal brain injury. Comprehensive neuropathological study was undertaken in 26 fatal patients. There was a clear rank order of the mortality rate in the lesion type. The rank order of good recovery and moderate disability was also similar to the inverse of the mortality ranking. The pathological "marker" of DAI, macroscopic lesions in the corpus callosum and dorsolateral quadrant of the upper brainstem and histological evidence of axonal retraction balls, were commonly found not only in patients with diffuse brain injury but also in focal brain injury. The type of intracranial lesion in severe head injury is thus an important factor in determining outcomes and DAI of varying severity is the common subjacent lesion in the fatal patients.

Keywords: Severe head injury; diffuse axonal injury; outcome.

Introduction

It is well known that the outcome of the patients with severe head injury is fundamentally dependent on the severity of impact injury, diffuse axonal injury[1, 7]. The type of intracranial lesion also has influence on the final outcome of the patients[3]. The present study was undertaken to investigate coexisting DAI and influence of the type of lesion on the outcome of severe head-injured patients.

Materials and Methods

The material included 107 patients with severe head injury all admitted to our hospital within 6 hours after head injury. They were divided into a group of diffuse brain injury (n: 44) and a group of focal brain injury (n: 63) according to their types of brain damage[3]. All patients had Glasgow Coma Scale (GCS) scores[3] of 7 or less on admission. They were further subdivided into four and three categories based on the principal findings on initial computerized tomographic (CT) scan. Diffuse brain injury was classified into DAI with classical features (n: 16), diffuse cerebral swelling (DCS, n: 8), massive subarachnoid haemorrhage in the basal cisterns (TSAH, n: 10) and nearly normal CT (n: 10). The mean age of the patients was 34 years. Focal brain injury was divided into traumatic intracerebral haematoma (ICH, n: 23), cerebral contusion with delayed haematoma formation (DICH, n: 14) and acute subdural haematoma (SDH, n: 26). The mean age of the patients was 48 years. The outcome of the patients was evaluated by Glasgow Outcome Scale[4] at three months after injury. Neuropathological study was undertaken in 26 fatal patients to identify the pathological "markers" of DAI, macroscopic lesions in the corpus callosum and dorsolateral quadrant of the upper brainstem and histological evidence of axonal retraction balls in the white matter.

Results

17 out of 44 patients with diffuse brain injury (38.6%) and 29 of 63 patients with focal brain injury (46.0%) had a score of 3 or 4 on the GCS on admission. The incidence of low GCS score was the highest in SDH (57.6%), followed by TSAH (50.0%), ICH (47.8%), DAI (43.8%), DCS (37.5%), DICH (21.4%) and nearly normal CT (20.0%). The overall mortality rate was 36.4% and the rate of good recovery was 11.4% in the patients with diffuse brain injury. They were 58.7% and 1.6% in patients with diffuse brain injury. There was a clear rank order of the mortality rates. The rate was the highest in TSAH, followed by SDH, DICH, ICH, DCS, DAI and nearly normal CT. The rank order of good recovery and moderate disability was also similar to the inverse of the mortality ranking (Table 1).

The age of 26 cases with neuropathological study ranged from six to 78 years and all patients sustained their injury in road traffic accidents. They lost consciousness immediately on impact and remained in coma until death.

The survival time ranged from six hours to 21 days. All patients with TSAH died within five days after head injury. 19 patients with focal and diffuse brain injury had signs of raised intracranial pressure manifested by pressure necrosis in one or both parahippocampal gyri. The macroscopic marker lesions and microscopic evidence of axonal retraction balls were commonly seen not only in

Table 1. *Lesion Ranking by Outcome*

Mortality				Good – moderate outcome		
Rank	Lesion type	% Dead		Rank	Lesion type	% G – M
1	TSAH	70.0		1	nearly normal CT	60.0
2	SDH	65.4		2	DCS	37.5
3	DICH	64.3		3	DAI	31.3
4	ICH	47.8		4	ICH	30.4
5	DCS	37.5		5	DICH	28.6
6	DAI	31.3		6	TSAH	10.0
7	Nearly normal CT	10.0		7	SDH	0

DAI: Diffuse axonal injury, DCS: diffuse cerebral swelling, TSAH: traumatic subarachnoid haemorrhage, ICH: traumatic intracerebral haematoma, DICH: cerebral contusion with delayed haematoma, SDH: acute subdural haematoma.

Table 2. *Distribution of Pathological Markers*

Type of markers	Diffuse brain injury (n: 10)			Focal brain injury (n: 16)		No. of cases (%)
	DAI	TSAH	DCS	ICH	SDH	
CC + DLQ + ARB	2	0	0	3	2	7 (26.9)
CC + DLQ	0	1	0	1	2	4 (15.4)
DLQ + ARB	0	2	1	1	2	6 (23.0)
DLQ alone	0	3	1	3	1	8 (30.8)
No lesion	0	0	0	0	1	1 (3.9)
No. of cases (%)	2 (7.7)	6 (23.0)	2 (7.7)	8 (30.8)	8 (30.8)	26 (100)

CC: Corpus Callosum, DLQ: Dorsolateral Quadrant of Brain Stem, ARB: Axonal Retraction Balls.

patients with diffuse brain injury but also in focal injury. Two or three "markers" were found in 11 of 16 patients (68.8%) with focal brain injury (Table 2).

Discussion

It has been reported that classical DAI is characterized by macroscopically focal lesions in the corpus callosum and dorsolateral quadrant of the upper brainstem and diffuse damage of axons[1, 7]. Blumbergs et al.[2] recently reported that the macroscopic lesions in the corpus callosum and the brain stem are only present in the brains in those patients with the most severe DAI. We could identify different degree of DAI in the majority of patients with focal brain injury. It is quite probable that patients with focal brain injury, associate with DAI. Sahuquillo-Barris et al.[5] also reported that this type of lesion is found

most often in SDH. But there was no difference in the incidence of "markers" between in patients with SDH and ICH. Pathological features of DAI were less common in patients with TSAH and DCS. The fatal cases with TSAH had quite a short survival time and may be associated with severe brainstem dysfunction[6].

DAI of varying severity is thus a common subjacent lesion in patients with severe head injury. But diffuse and focal brain injuries include multiple lesion types and the nature of them determines the final outcome of the patients with severe head injury.

References

1. Adams JH, Mitchell DE, Graham DI, Doyle D (1977) Diffuse brain damage of immediate impact type: its relationship to primary brainstem damage in head injury. Brain 100: 489–502

2. Blumbergs PC, Jones NR, North JB (1989) Diffuse axonal injury in head trauma. J Neurol Neurosurg Psychiatry 52: 838–841

3. Gennarelli TA, Spielman GM, Langfitt TW, Gildenberg PL, Harrington T, Jane JA, Marshall LF, Miller JD, Pitts LH (1982) Influence of the type of intracranial lesion on outcome from severe head injury. J Neurosurg 56: 26–32

4. Jennett B, Bond M (1975) Assessment of outcome after severe brain damage. A practical scale. Lancet 1: 480–484

5. Sahuquillo-Barris J, Lamarca-Ciuro J, Vilaita-Castan J, Rubio-Garcia E, Rodriguez-Pazos M (1988) Acute subdural hematoma and diffuse axonal injury after severe head trauma. J Neurosurg 68: 849–900

6. Shigemori M, Tokutomi T, Hirohata M, Maruiwa H, Kaku N, Kuramoto S (1990) Clinical significance of traumatic subarachnoid hemorrhage. Neurol Med Chir (Tokyo) 30: 396–400

7. Strich S (1956) Diffuse degeneration of the cerebral white matter in severe dementia following head injury. J Neurol Neurosurg Psychiatry 19: 163–185

8. Teasdale G, Jennett B (1974) Assessment of coma and impaired consciousness. A practical scale. Lancet 2: 81–84

Correspondance: Minoru Shigemori, M. D., Department of Neurosurgery, Kurume University School of Medicine, 67, Asahimachi, Kurume, 830, Japan.

Acta Neurochir (1992) [Suppl] 55: 40–42

Brain Oedema and Intracranial Hypertension Treatment by GLIAS

P. A. Oppido[1], **R. Delfini**[1], **G. Innocenzi**[1], **G. Di Giugno**[2], **J. Pecori-Giraldi**[3], **A. Santoro**[1], **M. Virno**[3], and **G. P. Cantore**[1]

[1] Departments of Neurosurgery, [2] Anaestesiology and Intensive Care, [3] Ophthalmology, Rome University "La Sapienza", Rome, Italy

Summary

The authors present their results regarding the use of a buffered solution of glycerol 30%-sodium ascorbate 20% (GLIAS) for the treatment of brain oedema and intracranial hypertension. GLIAS was perfused intravenously in 80 patients with several types of brain oedema. In every patients serum and urinary osmolarity, diuresis, main blood and urine parameters, and ICP were monitored. Following GLIAS infusion an increase in plasma osmolarity was observed, changing the average basal value plus 13.4% after 15 min., 10.5% after 30'. At the same time there was a reduction of ICP and improvement in cerebral compliance. In each case there was a decrease in intracranial hypertension and brain oedema without significant collateral effects.

Keywords: Glycerol; brain oedema; intracranial pressure; ascorbate.

Introduction

Brain oedema may accompany a wide variety of lesions resulting from head trauma, cerebral ischaemia, brain tumours, encephalitis, haemorrhages, systemic disorders or other injuries and disorders. Deterioration of brain function and progressive deepening of coma in acute neurologic emergencies is often a result of increased intracranial pressure (ICP) due to cerebral oedema.

Drug treatment of brain oedema and increased ICP consist of several types of drugs: diuretics, corticosteroids, osmotic tension reducers. The latter are often efficacious, however, if they are used over a long period, they may produce some side effects such as a rebound phenomenon, fluid and electrolyte disturbances, renal lesions[3]. Among the osmotic tension reducers glycerol has long been recognized as an effective tool against brain oedema. It may be administered either orally or intravenously. By the former route gastric irritation and emesis may occur, and by the latter route haematuria and haemoglobinuria[5, 7].

In 1966 Cantore and Virno[8] demonstrated that, adding sodium ascorbate to a solution of high dose glycerol, the risk of haematuria and haemoglobinuria decreased, and the glycerol increased its efficacy for reducing ICP. Unfortunately, this was not a buffered solution because of the inconstant sodium ascorbate pH. In fact they were only able to make extemporaneous solutions, which were difficult to use in clinical practice. Only in the last 2 years we were able to administer intravenously a buffered and steady solution of glycerol 30% plus sodium ascorbate 20% (GLIAS) (Table 1), to patients with brain oedema. We examined the clinical pharmacology of GLIAS and its efficacy in reducing ICP.

Table 1. *Population Studied*[*]

	Cases
Peritumoral oedema	10
Post-traumatic oedema	16
Post-operative oedema	21
Intraoperative oedema	28
Brain protection during vascular surgery	15

[*] According to different intracranial disorders.

Materials and Methods

We studied 80 patients, 36 male and 44 female, ranging in age from 12 to 79 years (average 46.7 y.), with several intracranial diseases: brain tumours, brain injuries, intracerebral haemorrhages, cerebral aneurysms, and other space-occupying lesions.

GLIAS was perfused as intermittent intravenous boluses for the treatment of different types of brain oedema and for brain protection (Table 2) according to 3 dose patterns:

1) Chronic Dosage: 0.7 ml/kg i. v., equivalent to 0.21 gm/kg glycerol and 0.14 gm/kg sodium ascorbate, every 6 hr. per day, for 3 days on average;

2) Intra-operative Dosage: 1.4 ml/kg i. v., equivalent to 0.42 mg/kg glycerol and 0.28 gm/kg sodium ascorbate during the craniotomy;

3) Brain Protection Dosage: 1.4 ml/kg GLIAS i. v., plus 250 mg phenytoin i. v. and 300 mg vit. E i. m., before temporary clipping.

The following parameters were monitored before and after GLIAS administration: haematochemical data, blood gases, urinary data, serum and urinary osmolarity, serum and urinary electrolytes, hourly diuresis, blood pressure and ICP. Serum osmolarity was examined in blood samples obtained before and 5', 15', 30', 60', and 180' min. after the start of the infusion. In patients undergoing chronic treatment the serum osmolarity was analyzed every day. The ICP monitoring was always made using Camino fiber optic pressure transducer n. 4 French[*]. During intra-operative GLIAS infusion intraparenchymal ICP was recorded[2] through the first burr hole of the craniotomy.

Table 2. *Composition of GLIAS Solution*

GLIAS solution (100 ml)	
Glycerol	30 gm
Sodium ascorbate	20 gm
Tioglycerol	0.2 gm
pH	7.4
Osmolarity	5007 mOsm/l[*]
Caloric Iitake	129.6 cal/100 ml

[*] Mannitol 18%: 1124 mOsm/l

Results

After administration of GLIAS we observed an increment in plasma osmolarity with respect to base values of approximately 13.5% after 15', 10.4% after 30', 6.1% after 60', and 4.8% after 180' min (Fig. 1). Base values returned after a period varying from 4 to 6 hours. These data (Fig. 1) demonstrate that GLIAS produces a more intense and prolonged plasma osmolarity than glycerol 10% and mannitol 18%[3]. In surgical patients, after GLIAS infusion, brain debulking was macroscopically evident on opening the dura mater and was, in all cases, adequate for surgical management.

ICP monitoring showed a slight and transient increase of pressure in the first 5 minutes after the start of infusion, immediately followed by a clear improvment of cerebral compliance and a reduction of ICP with respect to base values.

---

[*] Camino Laboratories, San Diego (CA), U.S.A.

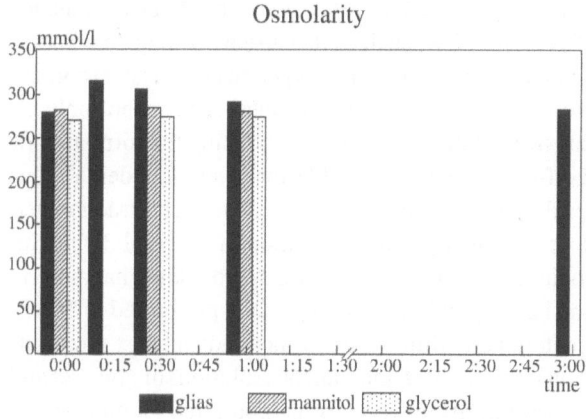

Fig. 1. Intracerebral pressure monitoring after administration of GLIAS, manitol or glycerol. Horizontal axis: time in hours. Vertical axis: osmolarity in mmol/l

Urine output rate was about 2800 cc/24 hr. on average, without any disturbances of fluid and electrolyte balance, even after prolonged treatment.

There were no significant variations in natriaemia and mild hypopotassiaemia occured in only 6 cases (7.5%) within 24 hours of infusion that did not appear to be related to the duration of treatment.

In only one case haematuria occured after administration of 270 cc of GLIAS over 12 hours period; this disappeared on reducing the dosage. Haemoglobinuria did not occur in any of the patients studied nor there was any case of phlebothrombosis.

Discussion

The efficacy of glycerol in treating cerebral oedema has long been claimed, even in comparison to other osmotics[1, 4, 5]. Some authors report that glycerol reduces ICP more drastically and for a longer period than mannitol or even urea. As compared to these, glycerol also has a lower risk of rebound because it is metabolized by the cell by means of of Krebs' cycle and aerobic glycolysis[6]. On the other hand its use has always been limited for the haematuria and haemoglobinuria that it frequently causes. GLIAS, the osmotic solution used in this study, has the advantage of being exempt from these side-effects because it contains sodium ascorbate[8] which stops haemoglobinuria by reducing the osmotic gradient between erythrocyte and serum, increased by the accumulation of glycerol within the cell and consequent haemolysis. Further, it avoids haematuria by facilitating and thus impeding vasoconstriction of the afferent glomerular arterioles induced by the glycerol. At the same time the GLIAS solution retains all the advantages of glycerol 30%, such as its capacity to reduce cerebral oedema and intracranial hypertension. The ascorbate present in GLIAS potentiates these effects, not only by favouring diuresis but also by reducing the formation of the free radicals responsible for cerebral oedema[9]. Our results show that it is possible to administer fractionated doses of this hypertonic solution of glycerol 30% with sodium ascorbate 20% without provoking haematuria and haemoglobinuria. In their study performed in 1966[8], Cantore and Virno reported these advantages after administration of extemporaneous solutions of glycerol and ascorbate, but only recently has a buffered solution, stable at pH 7.4, become commercially available. In fact, the instability of the ascorbate meant that the solution had to be prepared immediately before i. v. infusion, with considerable drawbacks in clinical practice.

The high osmolarity of GLIAS (5007 mOsm/l), even with respect to mannitol 18% (1124 mOsm/l) and glycerol 10%, explains the rapid and prolonged increase in plasma osmolarity in all our patients, free of any side-effects. In none of our cases did the rebound phenomenon occur, even at chronic doses, because the glycerol can be metabolized by the cell according to the mechanism mentioned previously. In fact, GLIAS has its own caloric intake (129,6 cal/100ml) contrary to the other osmotics, without altering normal glucide metabolism. Changes in hydro-electric balance were always kept well under control even during chronic treatment.

ICP monitoring confirmed that GLIAS is able to reduce ICP and improve cerebral compliance, with the typical ICP recording of glycerol: slight and transient increase of ICP in the first few minutes during infusion due to increased cerebral blood volume, followed by a progressive reduction[4]. Intra-operative infusion always provided sufficient brain debulking for surgical management. Experience with GLIAS during neurosurgical vascular surgery in order to provide, together with phenytoin and Vit. E, brain protection proved positive. However, this study was based on an insufficiently large number of patients to confirm a significance of the results obtained, but they have encouraged us to continue our studies with the use of GLIAS for brain protection. GLIAS was also found to have greater osmotic activity with respect to glycerol 10% and mannitol 18%, producing a more intense and prolonged plasma osmolarity, without significant side-effects and, overall, without causing the haemoglobinuria and haematuria so frequent after chronic treatment or with glycerol 10%, nor the hydro-electric alterations or the rebound phenomenon commonly observed after prolonged treatment with mannitol 18%.

References

1. Cantore GP, Guidetti B, Virno M (1964) Oral glycerol for the reduction of intracranial pressure. J Neurosurg 21: 278–283
2. Crutchfield JS, Narayan RK, Robertson CS, Lloyd HM (1990) Evaluation of a fiber optic intracranial pressure monitor. J Neurosurg 72: 482–487
3. Di Giugno G, Rosa G (1984) Modificazioni idroelettrolitiche da diuretici osmotici e furosemide, utilizzati nel trattamento della ipertensione endocrina. Min Anest 50: 482–487
4. Garcia-Sola R, Gilsonz F, Chillon D (1989) Immediate and long term effects of mannitol and glycerol: a comparative experimental study. In: JT Hoff *et al* (eds), Intracranial pressure VII. Springer, Berlin Heidelberg, pp 451–453
5. Pitlich WH, Pirikitakuihir P, Painter MJ, Wessel HP (1982) Effects of glycerol and hyperosmolarity on intracranial pressure. Clin Pharmacol 31: 466–471
6. Tao RC, Nelly RE, Yashimura NN, Benjamin F (1985) Glycerol: its metabolism and use as intravenous energy source. JPEN 7: 479–488
7. Tourtellotte WW, Reinglass JL, Newkirk TA (1971) Cerebral dehydration action of glycerol. Historical aspects with emphasis on toxicity and intravenous administration. Clin Pharmacol Ther 13: 159–171
8. Virno M, Della Rocca L, Pecori-Giraldi J, Cantore GP (1966) Scomparsa dell'ematuria provocata dal glicerolo endovenoso nel coniglio mediante associazione glicerolo-ascorbato di sodio. Gazz Int Med Chir 51: 256–267
9. Yukio I, Donlin ML (1990) The molecular basis of brain injury and brain edema: the role of oxygen free radicals. Neurosurgery 27: 1–11

Correspondence: Dr. P. A. Oppido, Department of Neurosurgery, Universita "La Sapienza", Viale Ippocrate n. 104, 00161 Roma, Italy.

Acta Neurochir (1992) [Suppl] 55: 43–46

Sedatives and Antagonists in the Management of Severely Head-Injured Patients

R. L. Chiolero[1] and **N. de Tribolet**[2]

[1] Department of Anesthesia, [2] Department of Neurosurgery, Centre Hospitalier Universitaire Vaudois, Lausanne, Switzerland

Summary

Continuous intravenous sedation is often prescribed during the intensive treatment of severe head injury. It is known that intravenous hypnotics may prevent or treat the brief intracranial hypertension episodes associated with nociceptive stimuli, like tracheal intubation. However there is yet no clear evidence in the literature showing beneficial effects of sedation in severely head-injured patients on intracranial pressure control or outcome. Sedation should be primarily administred in neurotraumatology to allow good conditions for intensive treatment, while avoiding any depressive cardiovascular action. The abrupt reversal of sedation by means of specific antagonists may induce significant elevation of both cerebral blood flow and intracranial pressure and should be avoided.

Keywords: Sedatives; barbiturates; benzodiazepines; flumazenil; head injury.

Role of Sedation in Neurotraumatology

The aim of intensive medical treatment of severely head-injured patients is to provide conditions favouring the recovery of brain tissue and to prevent secondary cerebral damage due to elevated intracranial pressure (ICP), systemic hypotension, hypercarbia and hypoxaemia. Pain and nociceptive stimuli, such as endotracheal tube mobilization and chest physiotherapy may induce increases in ICP in patients with low cerebral compliance and induce a secondary decrease in cerebral perfusion pressure[8]. Hypnotics, opiates and muscular relaxants are usually administred to provide good conditions for mechanical ventilation by avoiding fighting against the ventilator and concomitant intracranial hypertension. Furthermore, it has been shown that the intravenous administration of barbiturates and other hypnotics may prevent or treat the brief intracranial hypertension episodes associated with nociceptive or painful stimuli like tracheal intubation[20]. As the ICP level has been shown to be a powerful predictor of outcome in severely head

injured patients, most protocols of intensive care include intravenous hypnotics or sedatives. However when considering the effects of these agents on ICP control and on the outcome of head injury, things are not that simple, as shown by the contradictory results of recent studies. Uncontrolled studies have shown favourable effects of barbiturates on ICP control[17], while positive effects were not found in three controlled studies (Table 1)[18, 21, 4].

Schwarz et al. compared the effects of mannitol and pentobarbital in a randomized study of 59 severely head injured patients with intracranial hypertension refractory to conventional treatment[18]. They found that mannitol was better than pentobarbital for ICP control. In addition, the outcome was not improved by barbiturate therapy; in patients without intracranial haematoma, pentobarbital administration was associated with a worse outcome. Ward et al. evaluated the effects of prophylactic pentobarbital administration in head-injured patients with either intradural haematomas requiring surgical decompression or without mass lesion but whose best motor response was abnormal flexion or extension[21]. Barbiturates improved neither the outcome nor the incidence of elevated ICP. Eisenberg et al. studied the effects of pentobarbital therapy in a five-center randomized study on 73 patients with intracranial hypertension refractory to maximal conventional therapy[4]. The results indicated a 2:1 benefit on ICP control for those patients receiving barbiturates. It was not possible to evaluate the effect on outcome due to cross over of some patients in the conventional therapy. The results of these studies do not provide convincing evidence for a particular treatment of severely head-injured patients, although these agents may help to control ICP in subgroups of patients with refractory intracranial hypertension. However, it can be argued that arterial hypotension, which occured in a

Table 1. *Effects of Barbiturate Treatment on ICP and Outcome in Head Injury*

	Schwarz 1984	Ward 1985	Eisenberg 1988
Patients	59	53	73
Inclusion	Elevated ICP	Operated IDH	Elevated ICP
Criteria		Flexor/extensor Posturing	
Study	Prophylactic	Prophylactic	Therapeutic
Comparison	Pentobarbital vs Mannitol	Stand.Tretment +/− Pentobarbital	Stand.treatment +/− Pentobarbital
ICP control	Mannitol better than pentobarbital	No effect	Improved (2:1 effect)
Outcome	No positive effect increased mortality in pats without hematoma	No effect	Not evaluated
Side effects	Hypotension	Hypotension	Hypotension

* Four patients lost to follow-up.
IDH = Intradural Haematoma.

significant number of patients in the three studies, may have reduced the benefits of treatment.

Non-barbiturate sedative agents like midazolam and propofol are now avaible which allow good sedation, without inducing major systemic effects[16, 19]. However, as with barbiturates, there is yet no convincing controlled study demonstrating beneficial effects of these agents on ICP control and outcome in patients with severe head injury. Thus, even if it is often claimed that the main goal of sedation in neurotraumatology is to improve the control of ICP, the data presently available in the literature do not clearly support this statement. Sedation should therefore be primarily administred to allow good conditions for intensive managment, while avoiding any systemic adverse effects, particularly on the circulatory system. The choice of sedative agents should be made accordingly.

Effects of Sedative Agents on Cerebral Metabolic Rate and Haemodynamics

The agents commonly used for continuous sedation in neurotraumatology significantly affect cerebral metabolic rate, cerebral blood flow and ICP. Barbiturates produce a dose-dependent decrease in cerebral blood flow, CMRO2 and ICP (Piatt). In high doses, there is burst suppression on the EEG followed by electrical silence. The maximal decrease in CMRO2 approximates 55%, and is associated with an iso-electric EEG[15]. The main problems noticed with high doses of barbiturates are related to their potent systemic adverse effects, mainly arterial hypotension and prolonged recovery. Etomidate produces similar effects as barbiturates on cerebral

metabolic rate and haemodynamics[13]. Its strong suppressive action on steroidogenesis makes it an unsuitable agent for prolonged infusion.

Midazolam is presently a widely used agent for continuous sedation in intensive care patients. It decreases both CMRO2 and CBF. However, this effect is limited to about a 30% decrease in these parameters and burst suppression cannot be achieved[13,16]. It has limited systemic side effects; systemic haemodynamics are well maintained, allowing for safe use as prolonged infusion in neurotraumatology. The duration of action is shorter than that of diazepam, allowing for a reasonable recovery time following prolonged infusion.

Propofol is a new intravenous agent, which produces barbiturate-like cerebral effects, including burst suppression and suppression of cortical electrical activity in high doses[19]. It has a short duration of action and produces a dose-dependent depression of the cardiovascular system. It has been shown to be a convenient agent for both the induction and maintenance of anaesthesia for intracranial surgery. Recent studies have evaluated propofol as an agent for continuous sedation in ICU patients on mechanical ventilation, including head-injured patients[1, 5]. Recovery was found to be rapid in most of these studies, usually between 10 min to 120 min and was significantly shorter than that following midazolam infusion. Herregods *et al.* compared the effects of fentanyl and propofol (24 hrs infusion) on cerebral haemodynamics in a randomized controlled study including 25 patients with severe head injury[10]. They found similar levels of ICP in both systemic blood pressure and cerebral perfusion pressure following a bolus dose of propofol; in four of the patients the cerebral perfusion pressure fell below

50 mmHg[9]. Thus, the cardiovascular effects of propofol in high doses or following bolus injection may constitute the most important adverse effect of this agent in neurotraumatology, which should be avoided in head injury complicated by systemic hypotension and cardiovascular compromise. Further studies are necessary to define the place of propofol in neurosurgical sedation.

Antagonism of Sedative Agents

The activity of benzodiazepines on the central nervous system is related to the GABA receptors complex[11]. Various specific and nonspecific compounds may antagonize the central depressant effects of benzodiazepines. Flumazenil is a specific antagonist which will directly antagonize the cerebral effects of these agents (Hunkeler). Various clinical studies have demonstrated its value in the diagnosis and rapid reversal of coma due to benzodiazepine overdose as well as in the managment of prolonged recovery following general anaesthesia[14].

Flumazenil does not exert any significant effect on cerebral metabolic rate or on CBF. In normal subjects, Forster et al. observed no significant effect of flumazenil or of the flumazenil-midazolam combination on CBF in a double blind study[7]. The effects of midazolam antagonism by flumazenil after intracranial surgery were recently evaluated by Chiolero et al. in 18 patients operated on for brain tumour[2]. Anaesthesia consisted of midazolam for induction and maintenance, associated with N2O, fentanyl and pancuronium as muscular relaxant. Surgery lasted 5.5 +/– 1.3 hrs. Flumazenil, 1mg iv in 5 min, produced a very rapid recovery: after 2 min, 14 patients (78%) opened their eyes while 13 obeyed orders (72%) and 5 were extubated; at 5 min, 15 patients obeyed orders (83%) and 11 were extubated. The only side effects were a progressive drowsiness requiring a second injection of the antagonist in 3 patients and transient systemic hypertension in 7 patients.

The same authors evaluated the effects of the reversal of prolonged midazolam sedation by flumazenil in 15 severely head injured patients on mechanical ventilation[3]. All the patients had a Glasgow coma score below 8 on admission and cerebral contusion on the CT scan, while 7 had intradural hematomas requiring surgery. Flumazenil, 1 mg iv, induced a rapid arousal in 5 patients leading to removal of the tracheal tube; in 3 patients, a partial arousal with fluctuating leveles of consciousness was noticed, while no obvious sign of recovery was observed in the remaining patients. ICP and cerebral perfusion pressure levels did not change significantly in the patients with stable normal ICP during the 6 hrs preceeding flumazenil administration (i.e. continuously below 20 mmHg). By contrast, severe and highly significant elevations of ICP were noticed in the patients with unstable ICP during the same period (i.e. occasionally over 20 mmHg), with parallel decrease in cerebral perfusion pressure. Mean ICP increased from a baseline level of 18 mmHg to 40 mmHg after 5 and 10 min. This study clearly showed that abrupt reversal from benzodiazepine sedation in patients with head injury may induce dangerous levels of intracranial hypertension and should be avoided. Animal studies produced more complete explanations on the mechanisms of this phenomenon.

Fleischer et al. studied the effects of acute midazolam reversal on CBF, CMRO2 and ICP in normal dogs on mechanical ventilation[6]. Midazolam infusion, 40 mg.kg-1, decreased both CBF and CMRO2 to 75% of baseline values.

Flumazenil administration returned CMRO2 and EEG to pre-reversal levels; both CBF and ICP increased rapidly to greater than pre-reversal levels, while mean arterial pressure decreased significantly. These studies demonstrated that acute reversal of benzodiazepine sedation is associated with rapid increases in CBF and ICP, that can be clinically significant in patients with decreased cerebral compliance. Flumazenil administration should therefore be avoided in patients with severe head injury.

Conclusion

The effects of sedation during the acute treatment of head injury are complex. There are yet no data in the literature clearly demonstrating a beneficial effect of continuous intravenous sedation on ICP control and outcome. Convenient agents should be short-acting and free of side-effects on the cardiovascular system. The abrupt reversal by means of specific antagonists should be avoided.

References

1. Aitkenhead AR, Willatts SM, Park GR, Collins CH, Ledingham IMcA, Pepperman ML, Coates PD, Bodenham AR, Smith MB, Wallace PGM (1989) Comparison of propofol and midazolam for sedation in the critically ill patients. Lancet 2: 704–709
2. Chiolero RL, Ravussin PA, Freeman J (1988) Utilisation du flumazénil (Ro 15-1788) après perfusion prolongée de midazolam en anesthésie pour chirurgie intracrânienne. Ann Fr Anesth Réanim 7: 17–21
3. Chiolero RL, Ravussin PA, Anderes JP, Ledermann P, de Tribolet N (1988) The effects of midazolam reversal by RO 15-1788 on cerebral perfusion pressure in patients with severs head injury. Intensive Care Med 14: 196–200

4. Eisenberg HM, Frankowski RF, Contant CF, Marshall LF, Walker MD (1988) The comprehensive central nervous system trauma centers. High-dose barbiturate control of elevated control of elevated intracranial pressure in patients with severe head injury. J Neurosurg 69: 15–23

5. Farling PA, Johnston JR, Coppel DL (1989) Propofol infusion for sedation of patients with head injury in intensive care. Anaesthesia 44: 222–226

6. Fleischer JE, Milde JH, Moyer TP, Michenfelder JD (1988) Cerebral effects of high-dose midazolam and subsequent reversal with Ro 15-1788 in dogs. Anesthesiology 68: 234–242

7. Forster A, Juge O, Louis M, Nahory A (1987) Effects of a specific benzodiazepine antagonist (Ro 15-1788) on cerebral blood flow. Anesth Analg 66: 309–13

8. Gibson RM, McDowall DG, Turner JM, Nahhas MF (1975) Clinical experience of a method of continuous intracranial recording in 50 neurosurgical patients. In: Lundberg N, Ponten U, Brock M (eds) Intracranial pressure II. Springer, Berlin Heidelberg New York, p 496

9. Herregods L, Verbeke J, Rolly G, Colardyn F (1988) Effects of propofol on elevated intracranial pressure. Preliminary results. Anaesthesia [Suppl] 43: 107–109

10. Herregods L, Mergaert C, Rolly G (1989) Comparison of effects of 24-hour propofol or fentanyl infusions on intracranial pressure. J Drug Dev [Suppl] 2: 99–100

11. Hoffman WE, Prekezes C (1989) Corsendonk Workshop, Benzodiapines and antagonists: Effects on ischemia. Journal of Neurosurgical Anesthesiology 1 (3): 272–277

12. Hunkeler W, Möhler H, Pieri L, Polc P, Bonetti EP, Cumin R, Scheffner R, Haefely W (1981) Selective anatgonists of benzodiazepines. Nature 290: 514–516

13. Michenfelder JD (1988) Non-barbiturate induction agents: benzodiazepines, ketamine and etomidate. In: Michenfelder JD (ed) Anesthesia and the brain. Churchill Livingstone, New York Edingburgh London Melbourne, p 123

14. O'Sullivan GF, Wade DN (1987) Flumazenil in the management of acute drug overdosage with benzodiazepines and other agents. Clin Pharmacol Ther 42: 254–259

15. Piatt JH, Schiff Jr, SJ (1984) High-dose barbiturate therapy in Neurosurgery and intensive care. Neurosurgery 15: 427–444

16. Reves JG, Fragen RJ, Vinik R, Greenblatt BJ (1985) Midazolam: pharmacology and uses. Anesthesiology 62: 310–324

17. Rockoff MA, Marshall LF, Shapiro HM (1979) High-dose barbiturate therapy in humans: a clinical review of 60 patients. Ann Neurol 6: 194–199

18. Schwartz ML, Tator CH, Rowed DW, Ross Reid S, Meguro K, Andrews D (1984) The University of Toronto head injury treatment study: a prospective, randomized comparison of pentobarbital and mannitol. Can J Neurol Sci 11: 434–440

19. Sebel PS, Lowdon JD (1989) Propofol: a new intravenous anesthetic. Anesthesiology 71: 260–277

20. Shapiro HM, Wyte SR, Harris AB, Galindo A (1972) Acute intraoperative intracranial hypertension in neurosurgical patients: Mechanical and pharmacological factors. Anesthesiology 37 (4): 399–405

21. Ward JD, Becker DP, Douglas Miller J, Choi SC, Marmarou A, Wood C, Newton PG, Keenan R (1985) Failure of prophylactic barbiturate coma in the treatment of severe head injury. J Neurosurg 62: 383–388

Correspondence: Dr. R. L. Chiolero, Deptartment of Anesthesia, Centre Hospitalier Universitaire Vaudois, Lausanne, Switzerland.

Acta Neurochir (1992) [Suppl] 55: 47–48

Indomethacin (Confortid®) in Severe Head Injury and Elevated Intracranial Pressure (ICP)

K. Jensen[1], **J. Øhrstrøm**, **G. E. Cold**, and **J. Astrup**

Departments of Neuroanesthesia and Neurosurgery, Århus Kommunehospital, Århus C,
and [1] Department of Anaesthesiology, Aalborg Sygehus, Aalborg, Denmark

Summary

In five head-injured patients with cerebral contusion and oedema in whom it was not possible to control ICP by hyperventilation and barbiturate sedation, indomethacin (Confortid®) was used as a cerebral vasoconstrictor drug.

In all patients indomethacin reduced ICP to below 20 mmHg for several hours. Studies of cerebral circulation and metabolism during indomethacin treatment showed a decrease in cerebral blood flow (CBF) at 2 hours. After 7 hours, ICP remained below 20 mmHg in three patients, and these still had reduced CBF. In two patients a return of ICP and CBF to pretreatment levels was observed.

In all patients indomethacin treatment was followed by a fall in rectal temperature.

Outcome scaling has not yet been perfomed, but all patients left hospital without neurological deficits.

The results suggest, that indomethacin is an alternative in the treatment of ICP-hypertension in head-injured patients.

Keywords: Cerebral contusion; indomethacin; vasoconstrictors; cerebral haemodinamics.

Introduction

Several studies in patients with severe head injury (HI) indicate that intracranial hypertension might worsen the outcome, especially when ICP levels above 30–40 mmHg are recorded. Other studies suggest that ICP-hypertension is the primary reason for death in about 50% of the patients with severe HI.

Controlled hyperventilation, barbiturate coma and manitol treatment are generally recommended in patients with threatening ICP-hypertension, but it is wellknown that these therapeutic measures may fail to control ICP-hypertension.

In experimental and clinical studies indomethacin, a prostanglandin inhibitor, acts as a cerebral vasoconstrictor and reduces CBF while the cerebral metabolism is unchanged. In this study the effect of indomethacin administered i. v. over a 7 hour period was documented by measurements of ICP, mean arterial blood pressure (MABP), CBF, arterio-venous oxygen content differences (A-VDO2), A-VD-lactate and rectal temperature before and repeatedly during treatment.

Materials and Methods

Five males, median age 31 (22–42) years were studied. On arrival CT showed compression of the ventricular system and basal cisterns and progressive oedema in all patients.

After CT-scanning and possibly surgical decompression a subdural screw was inserted for continous ICP monitoring. MABP was monitored intra-arterially. The patients were intubated orally, hyperventilated and sedated.

The aim of treatment was to maintain ICP below 20 mmHg and to ensure a cerebral perfusion pressure (CPP) of at least 70 mmHg. Dopamine was administered if necessary. In order to control ICP-hypertension all patients were hyperventilated ($PaCO_2$ mean 3.4 kPa) and were in treatment with pentobarbitone (50–100 mg/hour) for at least 12 hours, before indomethacin treatment.

rCBF was measured by the bedside with Novo Cerebrograph 10a with 5 dectore places on each side over the parieto-temporal regions. A catheter was inserted in the internal jugular vein controlled with x-ray. Blood samples were drawn at the time of CBF measurements to calculate $AVDO_2$ and AVD-lactate. $CMRO_2$ was calculated as the product of average CBF-15 and $AVDO_2$.

The CBF measurements were performed immediately before indomethacin administration and at 15 min, 2 h, 4 h and 7 during indometachin infusion.

Indomethacin was given as an initial bolus of 30 mg and as a continous infusion of 30 mg/hour for seven hours.

Results

In all patients the bolus injection of indomethacin was followed by a decrease in ICP starting 5–10 sec. after injection. The decrease in ICP lasted about 4–5 hours (Table 1).

15 min after bolus injection of indomethacin a decrease in CBF-ISI was found in four patients. At two

Table 1. *Studies of $PaCO_2$ (kPa), CPP (mm Hg), ICP (mm Hg), CBF-ISI (ml/100g/min), $AVDO_2$ (mmol/l), $CMRO_2$ (ml O_2/100 g/min), Arteriovenous Difference of Lactate (AVD (lactate), mmol/l), Lactate/Oxygen Index (AVD/lactate)/$AVDO_2$)and Central Temperature (°C)*

		−15 min	15 min	2 hours	4 hours	7 hours
$PaCO_2$	(kPa)	3.4 ± 0.3	3.3 ± 0.4	3.3 ± 0.5	3.3 ± 0.4	3.4 ± 0.4
CPP	(mm Hg)	80 ± 13	89 ± 15	85 ± 10	76 ± 6	72 ± 9
ICP	(mm Hg)	28 ± 3	17 ± 6*	21 ± 4*	18 ± 4*	25 ± 11
CBF-ISI	(ml/100g/min)	34 ± 9	29 ± 11	25 ± 9*	28 ± 7	27 ± 9
$AVDO_2$	(mmol/l)	2.5 ± 0.6	3.0 ± 0.4	3.1 ± 0.2*	3.0 ± 0.4	3.0 ± 0.9
$CMRO_2$	(ml O2/100ml/min)	1.9 ± 0.5	1.9 ± 0.6	1.8 ± 0.4	2.0 ± 0.3	1.8 ± 0.9
AVD (lactate)	(mmol/l)	−0.13 ± 0.03	−0.18 ± 0.04*	−0.08 ± 0.09	−0.09 ± 0.05	−0.10 ± 0.11
Lactate/oxygenindex	(LOI)	0.05 ± 0.01	0.06 ± 0.02	0.03 ± 0.03	0.03 ± 0.01	0.04 ± 0.04
Central temp. (°C)		38.6 ± 0.8	38.5 ± 0.7	38.1 ± 0.5*	37.6 ± 0.4*	37.3 ± 0.4*

The CBF studies were performed 15 min before and at time 15 min, 2 h, 4 h and 7 h during indomethacin treatment (30 mg i.v. followed by 30 mg/h for 7h). Mean values ± SD are indicated.

*$p < 0.05$.

hours the decrease was significant with a decrease from 34 to 25 ml/100g/min in mean values. The decrease in CBF was accompanied by an increase in $AVDO_2$. The level of $CMRO_2$ did not change significantly.

Within the treatment period a fall in rectal temperature from mean 38.6 to 37.3 was observed.

Presently, 1–6 months after the injury, all patients have left hospital without neurological deficits.

Discussion

In the present study the general recommendations for treatment of ICP-hypertension were observed. In spite of intensified hyperventilation and barbiturate sedation in all patients ICP-hypertension developed. In this situation indomethacin treatment seems to be an alternative.

In experimental as well as in clinical studies indomethacin increases cerebral vascular resistance (CVR), decreases CBF while cerebral metabolic rate of oxygen ($CMRO_2$) remains unchanged.

We found in accordance with other studies that the administration of indomethacin was followed by a reduction in body temperature. We found a significant fall in ICP within a few minutes and lasting several hours. A fall in CBF within 15 min were recorded. Overall there was no change in $CMRO_2$.

The results suggest that indomethacin has a direct vasoconstrictory effect on the cerebral vessels, and therefore may provoke ischaemia. This would be indicated by a further fall in $CMRO_2$ and a net production of lactate in relation to oxygen uptake. In no case did lactate oxygen

index (Lo1) increase above 0.08, which according to Robertson *et al.* (1989) is the limit for ischaemic infarction.

This preliminary report of a beneficial effect of indomethacin on ICP-hypertension, cerebral circulation and metabolism is promising. However, a number of questions concerning indomethacin therapy and its effects on cerebral haemodynamics are yet unanswered.

References

1. Dempsey RJ, Roy MW, Meter KL, Donaldson DL(1985) Indomethacinmediated improvement following middle cerebral artery occlusion in cats. Effects of anaesthesia. J Neurosurg 62: 874–881
2. Pichard JD, Mackenzie (1973) Inhibition of prostaglandin synthesis and the response of baboon cerebral circulation to carbon dioxide. Nature New Biol 245: 187–188
3. Rosner MJ (1987) Cerebral perfusion pressure: link between intracranial pressure and systemic circulation. In: Wood JH (ed) Cerebral Blood Flow. McGraw-Hill Book Company, pp 425–448
4. Sakabe T, Siesjö BK (1979) The effect of indomethacin on blood flow-metabolism couple in the brain under normal hypercapnie and hypoxic conditions. Acta Physiol Scand 107: 283–284
5. Saul TG, Ducker TB (1982) Effect of intracranial pressure monitoring and agressive treatment on mortality in severe head injury. J Neurosurg 56: 498–503
6. Wennmalm Å, Eriksson S, Wahren J (1981) Effect of Indomethacin on basal and carbon dioxide stimulated cerebral blood flow in man. Clinical Physiol 1: 227–234

Correspondence: Dr. K. Jensen, Aalborg Sygehus, DK-9000 Aalborg, Denmark.

Acta Neurochir (1992) [Suppl] 55: 49–55

Prevention of Post-Traumatic Excitotoxic Brain Damage with NMDA Antagonist Drugs: A New Strategy for the Nineties

R. Bullock[1], **Y. Kuroda**[2], **G. M. Teasdale**[1], and **J. McCulloch**[2]

[1] Department of Neurosurgery, University of Glasgow, [2] Wellcome Surgical Institute, University of Glasgow, Scotland

Summary

Excitotoxic mechanisms due to overactivity of the amino acid neurotransmitters glutamate and aspartate maybe responsible for brain damage after injury. In this review we examine ischaemia and shear injury, which are relevant to human head injury. The opportunities for treatment using glutamate antagonist drugs are discussed.

Keywords: Head injury; brain ischaemia; excitotoxicity; glutamate.

Introduction

Neuropathologists have shown that ischaemic brain damage is by far the most common cause of brain damage in patients who die after head injury[7] (Fig. 1). Furthermore, the incidence of this pattern of damage has not significantly decreased over the last 15 years despite improvements in pre-hospital care, transportation, early diagnosis and intensive care of head injured patients[8, 18]. When intensive monitoring techniques are employed to detect conditions which may cause ischaemic brain damage in stabilised head injured patients, episodes of severe hypoxaemia and hypotension are relatively uncommon[7]. This suggests that ischaemic damage may be occurring either within the first hour or two after head injury, or occurring due to mechanisms which are not associated with obvious episodes of hypoxaemia, or hypotension. The neuropathological studies from Glasgow have shown that up to 40% of those patients who demonstrate severe ischaemic brain damage after death had spoken at some time after their injury, and this suggests that at least in this group, the latter explanation is more likely[17].

Recently, strong evidence has become available that a new mechanism may be responsible for a proportion of the "ischaemic type" of brain damage which is seen after head injury. The purpose of this review is to present evidence in favour of this "excitotoxic" mechanism of damage in different animal models, relevant to head injury and to discuss the implications of this evidence for the future treatment of head injured patients, using pharmacological agents which are currently nearing the end of pre-clinical testing.

The Excitotoxic Mechanism

When supra physiological concentrations of excitatory neurotransmitters are presented to post synaptic receptor sites, rapid and prolonged depolarisation of the neuronal membrane occur resulting in increased electrical activity and ion flux across the cell membrane, such that potassium leaves and sodium and calcium enters the intracellular space[11, 12, 27, 28, 34].

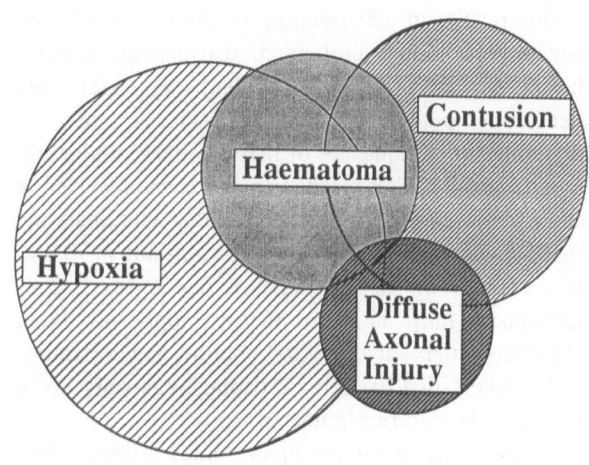

Fig. 1. Venn diagram to show the interrelationship of different pathophysiological processes responsible for brain damage in patients who die after head injury. Note that ischaemic neuronal damage is present in over 80%

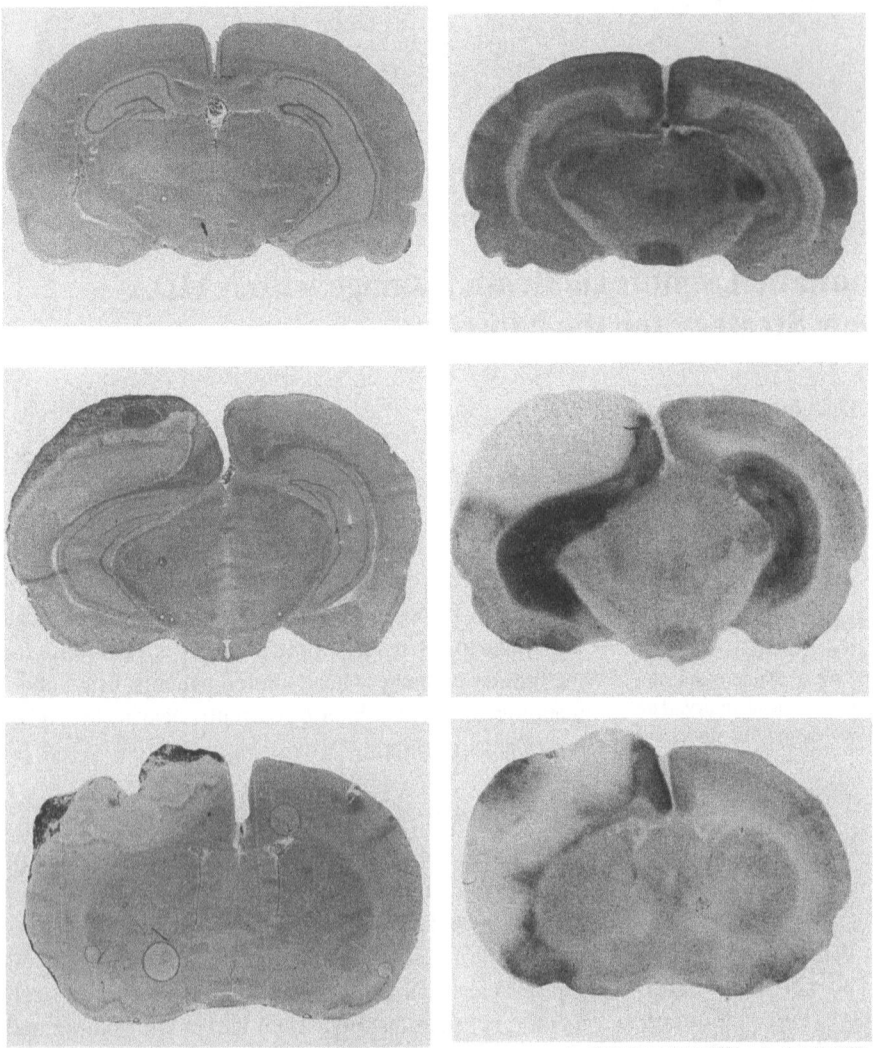

Fig. 2. Patterns of glucose hypermetabolism following acute subdural haematoma in the rat. Left: H and E stained brain sections. Right: 14C2D-oxyglucose autoradiograms (magnification × 10). Top row: Sham operated rat. Second row: Acute subdural haematoma – note the zone of pallor of staining beneath the subdural haematoma and corresponding reduction in glucose metabolism with peri-ischaemic hypermetabolism and marked hippocampal hypermetabolism. Third row: Subdural haematoma-section taken through the level the caudate nucleus – note marked zone of peri-ischaemic hypermetabolism within the cortex

This results in cell swelling (sodium chloride and water ingress) and if prolonged, also damage to cytoplasmic enzyme systems and second messengers, and release of potentially toxic substances such as polyamines (consequences of massive intracellular calcium release)[28, 34]. This mechanism has been most clearly shown for the excitatory neurotransmitters glutamate and aspartate which mediate synaptic transmission in 70% of the synapses in the mammalian neo-cortex[14]. This mechanism may also in theory apply to other neurotransmitters such as acetyl-choline, and dopamine.

It is likely that excitotoxic damage can only occur under certain specific circumstances:

1. When the glutamate uptake mechanisms which exist in the presynaptic terminal and in adjacent astrocytes has been inactivated so that concentrations of glutamate within the synaptic cleft over 2 micromolar can develop[1, 27, 32, 35]; there is evidence that glutamate uptake systems may not be fully active during certain phases of development of the immature nervous system and in tissue culture[13, 24]. Glutamate uptake is also inhibited by high concentrations of extracellular postassium[1, 11, 12].

2. When the post-synaptic neuron possessses sufficient energy reserves to be depolarised – i.e. when a resting membrane potential exists.

3. When high glutamate or aspartate concentrations are present in the synaptic cleft, either due to ischaemia or excessive functional or pathological depolarisation, as in seizures, for example.

The sensitivity of the glutamate uptake systems to different severities and durations of ischaemia in different parts of the nervous system has not yet been determined. There is a close relationship between the structures of the mammalian brain with the greatest sensitivity to ischaemic neuronal damage and the distribution of glutamatergic receptor sites (especially the N-Methyl-D-Aspartate (NMDA) receptor[11,14].

The origins of the increased extracellular glutamate seen in ischaemia have not been unequivocally established[1,11]. Studies with the microdialysis technique have shown that extracellular glutamate concentrations are massively increased (seven to twentyfold) in different circumstances of cerebral ischaemia, although glutamate release alone does not constitute conclusive evidence of an "excitotoxic" process: metabolic hyperactivation or an increase in electrophysiological activity must be also be shown[3,5,9,20,22,25,36].

When glutamate in very high concentrations is applied to the normal rat cortex, patterns of neuronal necrosis are produced which are indistinguishable from that caused by ischaemic damage alone[11,35]. Likewise the patterns of cell shrinkage and pyknosis which are produced when concentrations of about 100 micromolar glutamate are applied to neurons in tissue culture are similar to those seen when tissue culture cells are grown in severely hypoxic conditions[11,13].

Global Ischaemic Brain Damage

Brief, transient global cerebral ischaemia is probably very common after severe head injury. Studies with the Penn-I and Penn-II impact acceleration/deceleration model of head injury in the primate have shown that brief apnoea is an inevitable consequence of severe impact injury[15]. In many patients, concomitant chest injury and airway obstruction occur causing hypoxaemia[30]. Shock is also reasonably common when severe head injury is combined with multi-system trauma as is often seen after motor vehicle accidents[30,31].

Studies with microdialysis in animal models of transient global ischaemia have shown up to an 800% increase in the glutamate concentration in extracellular fluid which rapidly returns to normal levels when brain perfusion in restored[3] (Table 1).

In pilot studies with the microdialysis technique in head injured humans, high glutamate concentrations were shown to persist while raised intracranial pressure was present after a severe diffuse head injury[34].

Studies with the 2-Deoxyglucose autoradiographic method of measuring cerebral metabolism have shown a marked but transient increase in glucose metabolism in the CA_1 sector of the hippocampus especially, persisting for about two hours after global forebrain ischaemia in both rats and gerbils[16].

Mild transient forebrain ischaemia has also been shown to produce delayed neuronal death in the hippocampus, developing about 48 hours after the ischaemic period[23]. This results in complete pyknosis of neurons at about seven days after the ischaemic event, while neuronal morphology is normal to light microscopy within the first 24 hours. These patterns of delayed

Table 1. *Magnitude and Duration of Extracellular Glutamate Release Ischaemia/Trauma*

Species/model	Magnitude of glutamate release (site)	Duration	Investigators
Bilateral carotid occlusion and hypvolaemic hypotension – rats	800% (Hippocampus)	20 mins (10 mins ischemia with reperfusion)	Benveniste et al. 1984
Global transient* ischaemia – cat	approx. 700% (ischaemic cortex)	–	Shimada et al. 1989
Middle cerebral artery occlusion – rats	1,755% (ischaemic cortex) 2,750% (ischaemic striatum)	80 mins 90 mins	Butcher et al. 1991 (in press)
Subdural haematoma – rat	339% Hippocampus (non-ischaemic) 750% Ischaemic cortex	> 3 hrs 90 mins	Bullock et al. 1991 (in press)
Fluid percussion injury – rat	500% (impact site)	40 mins	Katayama et al. 1988
Weightdrop cord injury – rabbit	630% (impact site)	50 mins	Panter et al. 1989

*Bilateral carotid occlusion, coagulation of thyrocervical trunk.

neuronal death may have relevance after human head injury. Neuropathological studies have shown that ischaemic damage occurs in the hippocampus bilaterally in about 88% of patients who die after severe head injury[17].In over half the patients in whom no evidence of raised intracranial pressure can be demonstrated at any time during the clinical course or at post mortem, evidence of hippocampal ischaemic damage is present after death[17]. This may accord with the frequent memory and personality deficits which follow severe head injury in survivors.

Focal Ischaemic Damage After Head Injury and Excitotoxitcity

Severe focal ischaemic damage occurs in at least half of all patients with a major head injury[17, 18, 31]. We have performed tomographic cerebral blood flow mapping studies after focal head injury – (cerebral contusion and intracerebral haematomas) and have found zones of acute ischaemia around these lesions in every single patient studied acutely[6].

Post mortem studies have shown ischaemic damage to be common in the hemisphere underlying an acute subdural haematoma, and this accords with our results in a rat model of acute subdural haematoma[17, 29] (vide infra). In a few patients with severe head injury, vasospasm will develop in focal areas of the cerebral circulation, and in some of these, it may be sufficiently severe to cause infarction[26]. Evidence for this mechanism has been demonstrated by angiographic studies and more recently by studies using trans-cranial doppler[26].

Several studies have now shown that large amounts of glutamate and aspartate are released in the core of a focal ischaemic lesion such as following middle cerebral artery occlusion[9, 19] (Table 1). In our own studies, the magnitude of glutamate release was closely correlated with the size of the infarct, and glutamate levels had decreased by approximately one and a half hours after middle cerebral artery occlusion[19]. Shirashi and Simon have shown a zone of transient hypermetabolism for glucose occurring in a band at the periphery of the frankly ischaemic zone after middle cerebral artery occlusion in the rat and they speculate that this represents a zone of excitatory activity induced by glutamate release[36].

The most compelling evidence that glutamate induced excitotoxic mechanisms are responsible for a large proportion of the ischaemic damage in models such as middle cerebral artery occlusion comes from pharmacological studies with glutamate antagonists particularly the NMDA antagonists (Table 1) (vide infra).

Acute Subdural Haematoma in the Rat

We have recently devised a model of acute subdural haematoma in the rat which consistently produces a zone of focal ischaemic damage immediately underlying the thickest part of the haematoma which amounts to about 14% of hemisphere volume[29]. Studies of glucose metabolism have shown that the periphery of this ischaemic zone demonstrates a phase of transient hypermetabolism which persists somewhere between two and four hours after induction of the haematoma[20]. The most striking feature of this model, however, is the development of massively increased metabolism in both hippocampi (142% increase seen two hours after the haematoma in the ipsilateral Ca_1 sector) which has disappeared by four hours (Fig. 2)[20]. Using microdialysis techniques to measure levels of excitatory amino acids in this model, we have shown a sevenfold increase in glutamate and a fivefold increase in aspartate which peaks at about 20 minutes after the haematoma and which has normalised by one hour[5]. A threefold increase in glutamate release was seen in the ipsilateral hippocampus, a site at which cerebral blood flow was preserved ($\pm$ 95 ml^{-1}.100g^{-1}.min). These high levels of glutamate and aspartate were present throughout the three hour experiment in contrast to the brief peak seen in the focal ischaemic zones. These findings are strongly suggestive of a transient "excitotoxic" process which is possibly responsible for worsening the ischaemic damage under the haematoma and which may also render the hippocampus more vulnerable to other insults (vide infra). There is also evidence that ischemic damage in this rat model of subdural haematoma can be substantially reduced by the use of competitive glutamatergic antagonists (vide infra)[10].

Animal Models of Axonal Injury and Glutamate Release

It was generally believed that shear damage to axons occurs at the time of impact, to cause diffuse axonal injury. Such instantaneous mechanical damage would be irreversible and impossible to palliate. Recent evidence, however, challenges this concept. Blumberg and North have recently shown that up to a third of patients with severe diffuse axonal injury at post mortem had spoken at some tome after injury and prior to death suggesting possible secondary mechanisms[4]. There is also histological evidence to suggest that axon cylinders remain intact early after axonal shear injury and that disruption of the membrane maybe a secondary event dependent upon loss of axonal transport. There is thus, great interest in exploring concepts of secondary axon and neuron damage following shear injury to axons. Of the animal models which have been studied in the past, only the primate studies of Gennarelli and Thibault et al have accurately mimicked diffuse axonal injury in humans[15]. The fluid percussion injury model, although less relvant to human head injury, has yielded interesting results to suggest that glutamate release may be contributing to brain damage after shear injury. Katayama *et al.* and Panter *et al.* have used the microdialysis technique in rats with fluid percussion injury, and spinal cord injury. (Table 1)[22, 32]. These experiments have shown a surge in extracellular fluid glutamate levels to six to seven times higher than basal, immediately after the impact. These increases are transient, lasting less than one hour. Becker's group have also shown massive efflux of potassium associated with fluid percussion injury, consistent with brief depolarisation of neuronal membranes[2].

In other expriments with the fluid percussion injury model, Jenkins *et al.* have used a much less severe injury and studied its effect on memory performance in a radial arm maze[21]. These studies showed that animals treated with the non-competitive NMDA antagonist drug MK801 in an intermediate dose (1 mg/Kg) performed better after fluid percussion injury on the radial arm maze than did placebo treated controls, suggesting that the glutamate release occuring as a result of fluid percussion injury may be deleterious.

There is also evidence to suggest that the effects of fluid percussion injury may be synergistic with those of a mild ischaemic insult to cause an increased amount of brain damage[21]. Hayes and Jenkins *et al.* have studied rats with a relatively mild fluid percussion injury which was insufficient to cause axonal retraction balls. When a mild ischaemic insult (itself insufficient to cause neuronal damage) was added to this fluid percussion within one hour, the combined effects of both form of injury caused major ischaemic damage to appear in the hippocampus and areas of cortex when the animals were later perfusion fixed[21].

It is tempting to speculate that a mild ischaemic insult may be sufficient to inactivate glutamate uptake mechanisms in areas with a high density of glutamatergic synapses such as the hippocampus, so that glutamate released by the fluid percussion injury may then reach toxic levels, and damage cells, or predispose to damage. Such mechanisms may explain many of the phenomena seen in head injured patients, but hypotheses such as these require much more extensive study.

Table 2. *The Effects of Excitatory Amino Acid Antagonists in Experimental Focal Cerebral Ischaemia*

Species	Model	Agent	Pre-treatment/ post-treatment	Magnitude of neuroprotection	Investigators
Cat	MCA	MK-801	pre and post	− 50%	Ozurt *et al.* 1988, Park *et al.* 1988
	MCA	Ifenprodil/SL82-715	post	− 42%	Gotti *et al.*1988
	MCA	D-CPP-ene	pre and post	− 65%	Bullock *et al.* 1988
Rabbit	ACA/CC (temp)	Dextrorphan	pre and post	− 80%	Steinberg *et al.* 1988, 1989
Rat	MCA	MK-801	pre and post	− 41%	Park *et al.* 1988
	MCA	MK-801	pre	− 40%	Tamnura *et al.* 1988
	MCA/SHR	MK-801	pre	− 15%	Coyle, 1989
	MCA	MK-801	pre	− 54%	Bielenberg, 1989
	MCA/CC	MK-801	pre	− 73%	Buchan *et al.* 1990
	MCA	CGS 19755	pre and 5 mins post	− 63%	Simon *et al.* 1990
	MCA	MK-801	pre	− 45%	Lythgoe *et al.* 1990
	MCA	TCP	pre	− 27%	Gotti *et al.* 1988
	MCA	PCP	pre	− 55%	Bielenberg, 1989
	MCA	SL82-715	post	− 48%	Gotti *et al.* 1988
	MCA	Kynnuenate	pre and post	− 56%	Germano *et al.* 1987
	MCA/CC	Dextrorphan	post	− 53%	Kent *et al.* 1989
	subdural haematoma	D-CPP-ene	pre	− 54%	Chen *et al.* 1991

Neuroprotection was assessed histologically or with magnetic resonance imaging.

MCA = Middle cerebral artery occlusion, ACA/CC (temp) = temporary occlusion of anterior cerebral and common carotid, MCA/CC = middle cerebral and common carotid occlusion, SHR = Spontaneously hypertensive rats.

Table 3. *Excitatory Amino Acid Antagonists in Transient Global Ischaemia**

Species	Model	Agent	Pre-treatment/ post-treatment	Investigators
Gerbil	bilateral carotid occlusion	MK-801	1 hour before 5 mins ischemia 2, 24 hours after 5 mins ischemia	Gill *et al.* 1987, 1988
	bilateral carotid occlusion	CGS 19755	15 mins before 2, 4 hours after	Boast *et al.* 1988
		CPP	15 mins before 2, 4 hours after	Boast *et al.* 1988
Rat	bilateral carotid occlusion	CPP	15 mins after 10 mins ischemia	Swan *et al.* 1991
		CGS 19755	15 mins after 10 mins ischemia	Swan *et al.* 1991
		MK-801	15 mins after 10 mins ischemia	Swan *et al.* 1991
		MK-801	20 mins after 10 mins ischemia	Rod and Auer 1989
		Dextrorphan	15 mins after 10 mins ischemia	Swan *et al.* 1991

*Modified from Meldrum B[27].

The Effect of Drug Therapy on "Excitotoxic" Brain Damage – NMDA Antagonists

It is likely that future management of head injured patients will include multiple "neuroprotective" drugs – these may include calcium anatgonists, free radical scavengers and NMDA anatagonists.

NMDA antagonists have to date shown the largest magnitude of neuroprotective efficacy of any category of drug (Tables 2 and 3). These massive effects (up to a 64% reduction in the size of the infarct) have been seen with the competitive NMDA antagonist D-CPP-ene in a focal ischaemia model with pretreatment-middle cerebral artery occlusion in the cat. Evidence for neuroprotective effects is much less convincing in global ischaemia models, and some authorities dispute that these agents are effective at all after global cerebral ischaemia.

Conclusion

A major challenge facing clinicians who care for head injured patients is to identify those circumstances during the acute post injury course when excitotoxic mechanisms are most likely to occur, and thus to identify a window of "therapeutic opportunity" during which time these powerful neuroprotective drugs could be used. NMDA antagonist drugs may have significant side effects when used in doses which are neuroprotective, so that it seems unlikely at present that these drugs will be advocated for general use for all neurotrauma patients. Unfortunately, pathophysiological studies in various animal models have shown that the most important "excitotoxic phase" is probably maximal within the first few hours after injury[5, 27, 26].

Early diagnosis and optimal pre-hospital care, to minimise secondary ischaemic damage, therefore, still remains of paramount importance. Glutamate antagonist drugs may afford the opportunity to greatly reduce morbidity after severe head injury.

References

1. Anderson KJ, Monaghan DT, Bridges RJ, Travoularis AL, Cotman CW (1990) Autoradiographic characterisation of putative excitatory amino acid transport sites. Neuroscience 38: 311–322
2. Becker DP, Katayama Y, Tamura T, Gorman L, Cheung MK (1989) Excitatotoxic ionic fluxes and neuronal dysfunction following traumatic brain injury. J Cereb Blood Flow Metabol 9: 1: S 302
3. Benveniste H, Drejer J, Schousboe A, Diemer H (1984) Elevation of the extracellular concentrations of glutamate and aspartate in rat hippocampus during transient global cerebral ischaemia monitored by intracerebral microdualysis. J Neurochem 43: 1369–1374
4. Blumberg PC, Jones NR, North JB (1989) Diffuse axonal injury in head trauma. J Neurol Neurosurg Psychiatry 52 (7): 838–842
5. Bullock R, Butcher SP, Kendall, McCulloch J (in press 1992) Regional cerebral blood flow and extracellular glutamate release after acute subdural hematoma in the rat. J Neurosurg
6. Bullock R, Statham P, Patterson J, Teasdale GM, Teasdale E, Wyper D (1989) Tomographic mapping of CBF, CBV and blood brain barrier changes in after focal head injury using SPECT: mechanisms for late deterioration. In: Hoff J, Betz AL (eds) Proceedings of VIIth International Symposium on Intracranial Pressure and Brain Injury. Springer, Berlin Heidelberg New York, pp 637–639
7. Bullock R, Teasdale GM (1990) Head injury and brain ischemia: monitoring and prediction of outcome. In: Siesjo BK, Miller JD (eds) Proceedings of the International Symnposium on Brain Ressuscitation, Yamaguchi, Japan, 1988. Springer

8. Bullock R, Teasdale GM (1991) Surgical management of traumatic intracranial hematomas. In: Braakman R (ed) Handbook of clinical neurology, Vol 24. Head injury. Elsevier, Amsterdam

9. Butcher SP, Bullock R, Graham DI, MCCulloch J (1990) Release of neuro-excitatory amino acids from rat brain following middle cerebral artery occlusion. Br J Pharmacol 99: 277

10. Chen M-H, Bullock R, Teasdale GM, McCulloch J (in press 1992) Effect of glutamate anatgonist on reducing the ischemic damage after subdural hematoma in the rat. J Neurosurg

11. Choi DW (1990) Cerebral hypoxia: Some new approaches and unanswered questions. J Neurosci 10(8): 2493–2501

12. Choi DW (1987) Ionic dependence of glutamate neurotoxicity. J Neurosci 7: 369–379

13. Choi DW, Koh JY, Peters S (1988) Pharmacology of glutamate neurotoxicity in cortical cell culture: attenuation by NMDA antagonists. J Neurosci 8: 185–196

14. Cotman C, Monaghan D, Ottersen OP, Storn Mathieson J (1987) Anatomical organisation of excitatory amino acids receptors and their pathways. TINS 10: 273–280

15. Gennarelli TA, Segawa H, Wald U, Czernicki Z, Marsh K, Thompson C (1982) Physiological response to angular acceleration of the head. In: Grossman RG, Gildenberg PL (eds) Head injury: basic and clinical aspects. Raven Press, pp 129–139

16. Ginsberg MD (1990) Glycolytic metabolism in brain ischaemic. In: Weinstein PR, Faden AI (eds) Protection of the brain from ischaemia. Williams and Wilkins, Baltimore

17. Graham DI, Adams JH, Doyle D (1978) Ischemic brain damage in fatal non-missile head injury. J Neurol Sci 39: 213–234, 1978

18. Graham DI, Ford I, Adams JH, Doyle D, Teasdale G, Lawrence A, McLelland DR (1989) Ischemic brain damage is still common in fatal non-missile head injury. J Neurol Neurosurg Psychiatry 52: 346–350

19. Graham SH, Shiraishi K, Panter SS, Simon RP, Faden AI (1990) Changes in extracellular amino acid neurotransmitters produced by focal cerebral ischemia. Neurosci Letter 110: 124–130

20. Inglis FM, Bullock R, Chen MH, Graham DI, Miller JD, McCulloch J, Teasdale GM (1990) Ischemic brain damage associated with tissue hypermetabolism in acute subdural haematoma. Reduction by a glutamate anatgonist. In: Reulen HJ, Baethmann A, Fenstermacher J, Marmarou A, Spatz M (eds) Brain Edema VIII. Proceedings of the Eight International Symposium Berne, June 17–20, 1990. Acta Neurochir (Wien) [Suppl] 51: 277–279

21. Jenkins LW, Lewelt W, Young HF, Clifton GL, Hayes AL (1989) Muscarinic and NMDA receptor blockade attenuates increased post traumatic vulnerability to cerebral ischemia. J CBF Metabol 9: S750

22. Katayama Y, Cheung MK, Gorman L, Tamura L, Becker DP (1988) Increase in extracellular glutamate and associated massive ion fluxes following concussive brain injury. Neurosci Abstr 14: 1154

23. Kirino T, Tamura A, Sano K (1984) Delayed neuronal death in the rat hippocampus following transient forebrain ischaemia. Acta Neuropathol (Berl) 64: 139–147

24. Lucas DR, Newhouse JP (1957) The toxic effect of sodium L glutamate on the inner layers of the retina. AMA Arch Ophtalmol 58: 193–201

25. MacDermott AB, Dale N (1987) Receptors, ino channels and synaptic potentials underlying the integrative actions of excitatory amino acids. TINS 10: 280–283

26. Macpherson P, Graham DI (1978) Correlation between angiographic findings and the ischemia of head injury. J Neurol Neurosurg Psychiatry 41: 122–127

27. Meldrum B (1990) Protection against ischemic neuronal damage by drugs acting on excitatory neurotransmission. Cerebrovasc Brain Metabol Rev 2: 27–57

28. Michaels RL, Rothman SM (1990) Glutamate neurotoxicity in vitro: antagonist pharmacology and intracellular concentrations. J Neurosci 10: 283–292

29. Miller JD, Bullock R, Graham DI, Chen M-H, Teasdale G (1990) Ischemic brain damage in a model of acute subdural haematoma. Neurosurgery 27, No.3: 433–439

30. Miller JD, Sweet RC, Narayan R, Becker DP (1978) Early insults to the injured brain. JAMA 240: 439–442

31. Miller JD, Butterworth JF, Oudeman SK, Faulkner JE, Choi SC, Selhoust JB, Harbison J, Lutz HA, Becker DP, Young HF (1981) Further experience with the management of severe head injury. J Neurosurg 54: 289–299

32. Nichols D, Attwell D (1990) The release and uptake of excitatory amino acids. Trends Pharmacol Sci 11: 462-468.

33. Panter S, Yum SW, Faden AI (1990) Alteration in extracellular amino acids after traumatic spinal cord injury. Ann Neurol 27: 96–100

34. Persson L, Hillered L, Ponten U, Ungerstedt (1989) Intracerebral microdialysis for continuous metabolic monitoring of neurosurgical patients: preliminary methodological considerations. J Cereb Blood Flow Metabol 9: S 584

35. Rothman SM, Olney JW (1986) Glutamate and the pathophysiology of hypoxic ischemic brain damage. Ann Neurol 19: 105–111

36. Simon RP, Shirashi K (1990) N-Methyl-D-Aspartate antagonist reduces stroke size and regional glucose metabolism. Ann Neurol 27: 606–612

Correspondence: Mr. R. Bullock, University Department of Neurosurgery, Institute of Neurological Sciences, Southern General Hospital, Glasgow G51 4TF, U.K.

Acta Neurochir (1992) [Suppl] 55: 56–63

Posttraumatic Epilepsy in Civilians: Clinical and Electroencephalographic Studies[*]

A. Martins da Silva[1, 2], **B. Nunes**[1], **A. R. Vaz**[3], and **D. Mendonça**[4]

[1] Serviço de Neurofisiologia and [3] Serviço de Neurocirurgia, Hospital de Santo António, Porto, [2] Unidade de Fisiologia Humana and [4] Unidade de Biometria, Instituto de Ciências Biomédicas Abel Salazar, Universidade do Porto, Porto, Portugal

Summary

Posttraumatic epilepsy (PTE) is a known consequence of head trauma. The factors involved in posttraumatic seizures generation and the relationship between acute seizures and posttraumatic epilepsy are not without controversy. This also applies to the evolution of the electroencephalographic characteristics. The study here reported was performed analysing data from patients with posttraumatic epilepsy (N = 205) and data from patients followed-up since trauma and considered as a high risk population for the development of PTE (patients with acute seizures and/or patients with focal lesions – contusion, haematomas or penetrating head injury) (N = 152). Seizure type was associated with age and trauma severity (children, elderly and worst trauma cases present with a higher proportion of partial seizures). Neurological deficit and lesion location were associated with the seizure occurrence. The increased incidence of seizures was found when the most diffused brain dysfunction was combined with neurological deficits. The analysis of sequential EEGs performed at first, at 6th and 12 months post trauma revealed a non-stationary pattern throughout these time periods with EEG focal abnormalities remaining frequent for more than two years after the trauma. Children and old people have a higher proportion of EEG abnormalities with more frequent abnormal generalized activity in children and more frequent abnormal focal EEG activity in the elderly.

Keywords: Posttraumatic epilepsy; seizures; head trauma; electroencephalography.

Introduction

The impressive number of new cases of head trauma occurring every year caused by civilian accidents (traffic road, work and domestic) provide relevant data for investigating many aspects of neurological dysfunction. Posttraumatic epilepsy (PTE) is a known consequence of head trauma, and it is the major cause of non-idiopathic epilepsy only surpassed by congenital anormalities[4]. Out of the 500.000 patients/year head injured and hospitalized in USA, about 5.000 develop epilepsy[5]. These figures are of the most importance when age is taken into consideration. Head trauma was found as the major cause of neurological morbidity in children by Dusser *et al.*, 1989[2]. In our studies more than 70% of patients with PTE were less than 50 years old[8]. Worldwilde this morbidity and its inherent social consequences are afflicting large populations.

PTE has been well documented in many studies since Caveness and Weiss first introduced the notion that type and extent of lesion were important in the development of PTE. Studying soldiers they found that penetrating head injury was the most epileptogenic lesion[1, 17]. In the same type of population Salazar *et al.* found neurological deficits as factors frequently associated with PTE[6, 14]. Later studies by these authors progressed to the definition of cortical and subcortical structures involved[13]. In civilians, the studies of Jennet were the first to state the close relationship between skull fractures complicated by a torn dura and PTE[7].

PTE studies furnish many relevant features on different aspects of epileptology. PTE can be used as a model to study the evolution of seizures into a chronic stage of epilepsy. Experimental models based on mechanical induction of trauma[9] or on cortical implant of Fe derivatives[18] showed the importance of these factors and of cerebral parenchymal haemorrhage on PTE. Finally, meta-analysis of published data established interesting correlations between lesion location, lesion extension and PTE probabilities[3]. In spite of these results, many questions still remain unexplained. Examples of problems not solved are: i) the different time of seizure

[*] Work supported by JNICT (Portuguese Agency for Science and Technology) Grant 87183

onset and of seizure evolution in groups of patients with "similar" lesions; ii) the influence of immediate ressuscitation procedures and of acute intensive care on PTE. Other aspect not yet well documented is the lack of reliable prediction of long term neurological consequences, such as PTE. The study done by Walker, 1989 of 40 years follow up of war veterans is one of the few published with an extended follow-up. Besides these aspects the factors involved in the evolution of PTE may be different in acute versus late onset seizures and the consequences may also depend on the factors acting in isolation or together in the various phases of head trauma evolution. In addition to these difficulties, different studies have discrepancies in the conclusions, due to their heterogenous methodologies. The tendency to take for granted that some findings in war injuries may be applied to civilian accidents illustrates these discrepancies. The war injuries and civilian accidents have different neurological consequences because they cause different lesions: while penetrating head injuries (PHI) with prominent cerebral tissue loss are frequent in war traumas, closed head injuries are the most frequent type of trauma in civilian accidents. The same discrepancy on methodologies also applies to the different results obtained in the studies of prophylactic treatment for PTE prevention. In such studies discrepancies are related with the methodology applied, the different follow-up periods[12] or different populations samples[10] in the various series do not allowing definitive conclusions[15].

The value of electro-encephalographic (EEG) studies in the estimation of the risk for the development of epilepsy or in the estimation of the probability that the brain function returns to normality, in the function of trauma or patient characteristics, is also controversial. The relationship between EEG paroxysmal activity evolution and PTE has not been fully established in spite of the findings reported by Pampiglione, 1975. This author found relationships between trauma evolution, EEG and PTE when the analysis was performed 4 to 6 weeks after trauma[11]. However the long term evolution of such interrelationship, that is the relationship between EEG findings at different time intervals and outcome of severe head injury, is not well documented. The same author referred to the "appearance of discharges on EEG four or more months after the injury may precede the occurrence of clinically recognizable seizures". The difficulties of establishing any relationship between posttraumatic EEG findings and outcome of head trauma increase when age was taken into account as an associated factor[2].

The aim of the present study is to contribute to the discussion of some of the controversial aspects of head trauma due to civilian accidents. We studied the relationships between: i) head trauma and posttraumatic epilepsy; ii) head trauma and brain function (evaluated with sequenced EEG recordings); and iii) cerebral dysfunction, interpreted as EEG abnormalities, caused by head trauma and PTE. The study was performed analysing data from patients with posttraumatic epilepsy and data from patients followed-up since trauma considered as a high risk population for the development of PTE (patients with acute seizures and/or patients with focal lesions – contusion, haematomas or PHI). The beginning of PTE (seizure type, time of onset), its evolution, and the relevance of clinical and neurophysiological (EEG) variables on PTE, were studied.

Population and Methods

A group of 306 civilian head trauma patients was studied. It comprises two subgroups, one of which is the group of 154 patients who attended the outpatient clinic for epilepsy at the Hospital Santo António and studied retrospectively. They had a well documented history of head trauma after civilian accidents (mainly traffic road accidents) with epileptic seizures onset after the accident. The other subgroup refers to 152 head trauma patients admited to hospital during the years 1988 and 1989 and selected because of their potentially higher risk for developing PTE. Based on a review of the literature this increased PTE risk was defined as acute seizures (within 48 hours after trauma) and/or focal cerebral lesions (focal contusions, intracerebral haematoma or PHI). The prospective analysis was carried out on admission (or during the first month), at 6 and 12 months after trauma with clinical, EEG and CT scan examinations as a protocol design. The location of the lesion was determined by CT scan and in surgical patients confirmed by the neurosurgeon's report. At the time of data analysis (1990) all the patients from the first group had a minimum follow-up period of 5 years. In the prospective study patients had a minimum of one year of follow-up. Seizures (type, occurrence and time of onset) and their evolution were analysed as a function of the patients' age, trauma factors (type and location of the cerebral lesion, trauma severity defined by the Glasgow Coma Scale) and neurological deficits. The sequential EEG findings were also analysed as a function of trauma characteristics, seizures and longterm follow up.

Statistical analysis to test associations between categorical variables was performed using Chi Square Tests. The Kolmogorov Smirnov two sample test was used to compare the time elapsed between trauma and seizure onset according to the type of seizures (partial or generalized seizures). Logistic regression was applied to assess the combined effect of dominant factors on a dichotomic outcome variable (such as seizure occurrence: presence or absence of seizures within the first year of trauma).

Results

1. Seizure Analysis

The analysis of risk factors associated with the occurrence of seizures within the first year was performed on the 152 patients prospectively studied. Out of these 51 had seizures that occurred during the first year after trauma and the remainder had no seizures by the time of the analysis. The study of the relationship between type of seizure, the time elapsing between trauma and first seizure, and trauma factors was carried out in the whole group of patients with seizures (N = 205).

First Seizure: Time and Seizure Type

Time that elapsed between trauma and first seizure is shown in Fig. 1. It is interesting to note that in the retrospective study more than 25% of patients with seizures had their first seizure later than the first year after trauma. Partial seizures (P SZ), are more frequent – 54.6% – than generalized seizures (G SZ) – 37.6% – or the others types (7.8%). Restricting the analysis to the patients with seizures onset within the first year, the distribution of the number of days between trauma and seizure for patients with G SZ differed significantly from the corresponding distribution for patients with P SZ (p < 0.05). The cumulative distributions for patients with each type of seizures are compared in Fig. 2 (A and B). The frequency of G SZ occuring during the first 24 hours (55%) is higher than the frequency of P SZ (24.2%). Although P SZ are rising rapidly during the first week, by the fourth day the plots of the two cumulative frequency distributions become closer (56% of each type of seizure were present), and by the end of the first week the percentage of P SZ is higher than 75%. The plots by seizure type re-approach by the 6th month. These results also indicate that the highest proportion of P SZ occur between the 2nd and the 7th day.

Relationship Between Type of Seizure and Type of Cerebral Lesion

Restricting the analysis to patients with G Sz or P Sz and with lesions – PHI, focal contusion/intracraneal haematoma, and diffuse or hemispheric contusion (DC) – no significant association (either analysing the whole population with seizures or only those included in the retrospective study) was found between the type of Sz and type of cerebral lesion, although Psz seemed to be more frequent in patients with focal lesions.

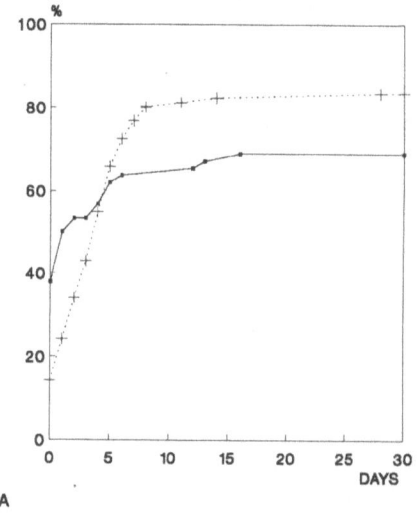

A

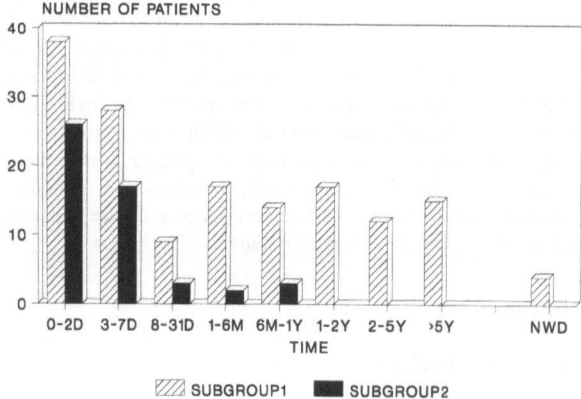

Fig. 1. Time of occurrence: first seizure. Patients with seizures N = 205

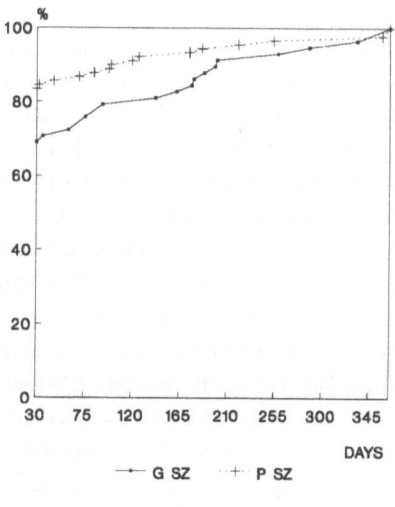

B

Fig. 2. Cumulative distribution of time between trauma and seizure by type of seizure. A) First month. B) One month-one year

Relationship Between Seizures Occurrence, Type of Seizures and Lesion Location

The relationship between seizure occurrence and lesion location (frontal, temporal, parietal, occipital, hemispheric, multiple or diffuse) was analysed in the patients prospectively studied. Figure 3 displays for each lesion location the frequency of each outcome as well as the proportion of patients with seizures. Temporal, parietal, hemispheric or diffuse lesions present higher percentage of seizures. However the seizure type is not related to the lesion location.

In order to proceed with the study of the relationship between lesion location and seizure occurrence the locus of the lesion was classified as focal and non-focal. These groups were organized as a function of the most relevant neurological lesion, as follows: one patient with focal temporal contusion and moderate generalized cerebral contusion was classified as having a focal lesion. Patients with severe cerebral contusion and intracerebral haematoma were included as non-focal lesions. A statistically significant association (p < 0.01) was found between seizure occurrence within the first year after trauma and lesion location: a much higher percentage of patients presenting with non focal lesions developed seizures when compared to the remaining patients. Among the patients with focal lesions, seizures were more frequent in those with parietal and temporal lesions.

Relationship Between Seizures Occurrence, Type of Seizures and Severity of Trauma

Severity of trauma defined according to the 15 points of Glasgow Coma Scale (GCS) was grouped into three different subgroups, in function of coma severiry: < = 7 GCS points, 8–12 points and > = 13 points. A significant association (p<0.001) was found between the type of Sz and the severity of trauma with a substantially lower proportion of Gsz on GCS < = 7 group and a higher proportion in the GCS > = 13. As it is shown in Fig. 4, 35% of the Psz occurred in the population with lowest GCS and 9.8% of Gsz belong to this GCS group.

Studying the occurrence of seizures during the first year it seems that the proportion of patients with a seizure increases as the severity of trauma increases. In the group with GCS equal or less 7 points the percentage of patients with seizures was 50%. This percentage drops to 36.7 and 24.8% respectively, for patients with GCS scores between 8 and 12 points, and higher than 12 points.

When analyzing seizure occurrence in relation to severity of trauma and lesion location (focal or non focal)

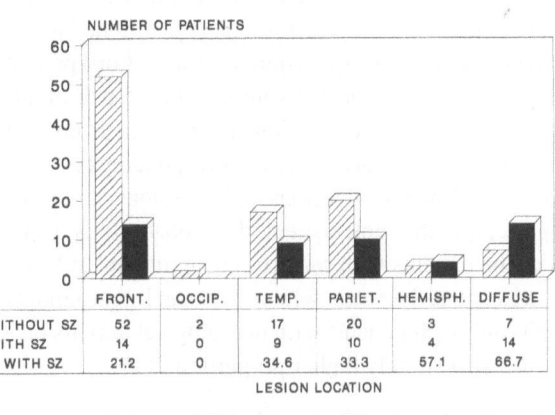

	FRONT.	OCCIP.	TEMP.	PARIET.	HEMISPH.	DIFFUSE
WITHOUT SZ	52	2	17	20	3	7
WITH SZ	14	0	9	10	4	14
% WITH SZ	21.2	0	34.6	33.3	57.1	66.7

Fig. 3. Seizures and lesion location

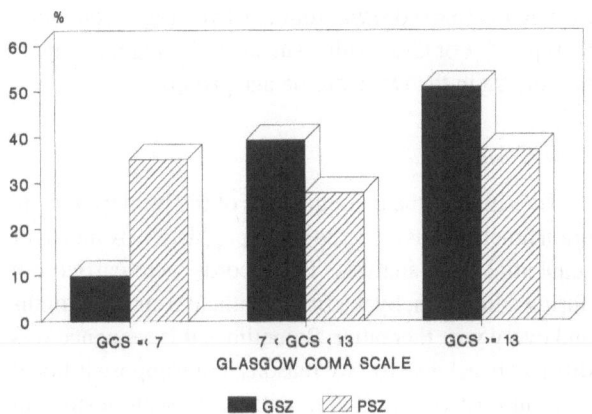

Fig. 4. Seizure type and severity of trauma

this latter factor remains significantly associated with seizures occurrence.

Relationship Between Seizures Occurrence, Type of Seizure and Neurological Deficits

Occurrence of seizures was significantly associated with neurological deficits (p < 0.001). Nearly 53.3% of the patients with neurological deficits developed seizures during the first year after trauma. The corresponding proportion for patients without neurological deficits drops to 25%. This strong association between neurological deficits and occurrence of seizures within the first year remains when the factor, severity of trauma, is also included in the analysis. Considering simultaneously the two factors: neurological deficits and local of lesion (focal/non focal), both factors remained statistically significant in determining its occurrence. According to this two factor model the predicted probability of having a seizure within the first year for a patient who had a non focal lesion and neurological deficits is 0.79. For a patient presenting a focal lesion and without clinical neurological deficits it is 0.19. For a patient having no neurological deficits and a non focal lesion the corresponding probability is 0.53. When focal lesions and neurological deficits are present, in the same patient, the probability is 0.44.

For the patients with seizures no significant association was found between seizure type and neurological deficits although patients with neurological deficits presented with a slightly higher proportion of PSz.

Relationship Between Type of Seizures and Age Groups

The relationship between Sz type and patients age was studied considering 5 age groups: < = 10, 11–17, 18–40, 41–60 and > 60 years old. A statistically significant association ($p < 0.05$) was found between age groups and Sz type (Psz or Gsz) with a substantially higher proportion of Psz in the two extreme age groups.

2. EEG Analysis

The study of the consequences of the head trauma on brain function was assessed in our population by means of sequential EEG analysis. The records were carried out during admission, by the first month, at 6 and 12 months and every year thereafter. Sometimes this sequence was difficult to achieve for two reasons: i) the impossibility of recording EEGs in patients with acute scalp lesions or recently operated upon. ii) the patients' acceptability of long follow up; patients without neurological or medical consequences although easily followed up at 6 or 12 months after the trauma fail later controls. For these reasons more than 75% of sequenced EEG studies have been carried out in the prospective group and the number

of patients studied at each time interval was different. The analysis was carried out by comparing the results at 1, 6 and 12 months.

Evolution of EEG Paroxysmal Activity

The 476 EEGs recorded from 259 patients at different time intervals after the head trauma were analyzed. The EEGs recorded at each time interval and their characteristics (Normal, Focal and Non focal activity) are shown in Table 1. The percentage of normal EEGs is 3.8% by the first week, increases markedly by the first month (30.4%) and reaches the value of 35.5% at one year. The small change in the proportion of normal EEGs is partially due to the small number of patients without neurological problems being followed-up 1 year after the trauma. Well defined EEG focal paroxysmal activity is already present at the first week after trauma, remaining as the most relevant EEG abnormality on the followed-up patients. It is important to note that in patients with PTE and with an EEG recorded two years or later after trauma focal abnormalities are higher than 60%.

The evolution of paroxysmal activity was studied in patients with EEGs recorded at one and six months (39 patients), one and twelve months (26 patients) and at six and twelve months (49 patients) after trauma. The percentage of unchanged EEGs, remaining normal or presenting the same pattern, is around 50% at the three different periods (1–6 months; 6 months–1 year and 1 month—1 year). Out of the patients with an initially normal EEGs 56.3% remained normal at 6 months and 70% at 12 months (Table 2). From the population with focal EEG abnormalities at 1 and 6 months, 66.7% and 56.5% remained focal at 6 and 12 months respectively. Out of the population with changed EEGs patterns, 37.5% of the normal EEGs at the 1st month changed to focal paroxysmal activity by the 6th month, and 31% of the normal EEGs at the 6th month moved to focal abnormalities at 1 year after trauma.

Table 1. *EEG Activity (at Different Follow-up Periods)*

Time of EEG recording	1–7 days	8–26 days	1 month	6 months	1 year	2 years	2–5 years	> 5 years
Normal	3.8	11.4	30.4	30.9	35.5	15.4	22.6	13.7
Focal	61.5	62.9	46.4	47.2	46.1	64.1	51.6	54.9
Focal and N focal	23.1	17.1	14.5	11.4	11.8	15.4	9.7	11.8
N focal	11.5	8.6	8.7	10.6	6.6	5.1	16.1	19.6
EEGs recorded	52	35	69	123	76	39	31	51

Table 2. *Evolution of EEG Paroxysmal Activity*

(%)—»	1 month – 6 months			6 months – 1 year			1month – 1year		
	Normal	Focal	N focal	Normal	Focal	N focal	Normal	Focal	N focal
Normal	56.3	37.5	0.0	53.8	30.8	7.7	70.0	20.0	0.0
Focal*	6.7	66.7	13.3	34.8	56.5	0.0	33.3	50.0	16.7
N focal*	0.0	66.7	33.3	0.0	16.7	50.0	0.0	0.0	50.0

*Low percentages of F + NF paroxysmal activity – not included.

Relationship EEG – Cerebral Lesion

At the first month, PHI and other focal lesions (focal contusion and intracerebral haemorrhage) had a very low percentage of diffuse abnormalities (6.3% and 7.9%), a relatively similar percentage of normals (37.5% and 31.6%) and a percentage of 37.5 and 47.4 of focal activity. By the sixth month the percentages of normal EEGs are almost similar for PHI and other focal cerebral lesion (30.7% and 28.6%) with increasing focal activity to 61.5% in PHI and to 49% on the other focal lesions. In the group of patients with hemispheric or diffuse contusions an equal percentage (44.4%) of normal EEGs and EEGs showing focal activity at one year after trauma was found. In this group of patients with hemispheric or diffuse contusions the percentage of normal EEGs increases with follow up (25% at one month and 44.% at one year after the trauma) (Table 3).

Relationship EEG – Trauma Severity

The relationship between EEG findings (normal, focal and generalized abnormalities) and trauma severity was assessed in terms of the 3 GCS groups previously described (< = 7; 8–12; > = 13). At the first month, in the group with GCS >=13, normal and focal abnormal EEGs have an identical percentage (35.3%). The percentage of EEGs with focal abnormalities in this GCS group increases up to 46.3% at one year records, while the percentage of normal EEGs is almost similar (31.7%). At the first month, the percentage of normal EEGs on group with GCS < =7 is low (9%) and the percentage of EEGs with focal abnormalities is high (63.6%). An increase in the percentage of normal EEGs (31.6%) and a decrease on the EEGs with focal abnormalities (42.1%) was found in this group by the 6th month. In the group of GSC > = 8 and < = 12 at one month the records show a higher percentage (59.1%) of EEGs with focal abnormalities, than of normal EEGs (31.8%). These values change at the one year records, increasing the number of normals (44.8%) and

Table 3. *EEG-Cerebral Lesion*

Cerebral lesion/ EEG activity		1 month	6 months	12 months
PHI	normal	37.5	30.7	40.9
	focal	37.5	61.5	40.9
	non focal	6.3	3.8	9.1
FC	normal	31.6	28.6	36.4
	focal	47.4	49.0	39.4
	non focal	7.9	10.2	9.1
DC	normal	25.0	35.7	44.4
	focal	37.5	35.7	44.4
	non focal	12.5	17.9	0.0

PHI: Penetrating head injury, FC: focal contusion and intracerebral haemorrhage, DC: diffuse contusion and hemispheric contusion. Percentages of F + NF paroxysmal activity not displayed.

decreasing the number of focal abnormal EEGs to the same percentage (44.8%). In summary and taking only the data at 1 and 6 months interval, the EEG evolution is different on the three GCS groups with increasing focal activity at 6 months (50%) in GCS > = 13 and an increasing number of normal EEGs in the other groups: 35% in GCS group 8–12 and 31.6% in GCS group < = 7.

Relationship EEG – Neurological Deficits

At the first month, in the group of patients with neurological deficits 66.6% have focal (F or F + NF) abnormalities, 14.3% non focal or generalized paroxysmal activity and 19% have normal EEG records. The percentage of normal EEGs increased up to 30.8% by the first year and of generalized paroxysmal activity decreased to 3.8%. In the patients without neurological deficits EEG focal abnormalities are also high (58.7%), but with a higher percentage of normal EEGs (34.8%). It is interesting to note that in both populations the focal abnormalities remained at similar values by the 6 and 12 months, nearly 60%.

Relationship Between EEG and Type of Seizures

At one month patients with Psz have a high percentage of focal (F or F+NF) EEG abnormalities (58.4%) and a low percentage of normal EEGs (8.3%). These values changed during follow-up with 33% of normal EEGs at 1 year after trauma. In patients with Psz, non focal paroxysmal activity drops from 33% at the first month to 5.4% and 9.5%, respectively at 6 and 12 months later. In patients with Gsz initial EEG focal abnormalities are also high (54.6%) but the percentage of normal EEGs (27.3%) is higher than in patients with Psz. There is an increase in the percentage of generalized activity in patients with Gsz from 18.2% at the 1st month to 25% at 6th month, and a decrease later (13.3%).

Relationship EEG – Age Groups

The relationship between age groups and EEG was studied at 6 months after trauma. It seems that the percentage of normal EEGs in children and aged patients is lower than in the other age groups. Furthermore, while children present the highest proportion of non focal activity, the aged patients showed the highest proportion of focal activity.

Discussion and Conclusions

The results presented here raise some points for discussion. Seizure analysis showed that partial or seizures partial at the beginning are the most frequent type of seizures in posttraumatic epilepsy notwithstanding their delayed onset. The proportion of each type of seizures is different on the first two days after trauma and thereafter. The generalized seizures are the first and the more frequent during the first days and the proportion of partial seizures is higher later. This is the first point open to discussion: the change in seizure type frequency. This change is probably related to the influence of different factors: influence of general factors on the generation of acute generalized seizures and of neurological involvement (neuronal damage) on non acute or later seizures. Nowadays, the general factors involved in the acute phase of trauma are more rapidly reversed by the resuscitation procedures and the cerebral lesions are for a shorter time agravated by hypoxic or other metabolic factors, decreasing the risk of generalized seizures and allowing a better characterization by patients and medical staff of the seizure type.

Apart from the acute factors the seizure frequency and seizure pattern is influenced by the evolution of the neuronal damage. The clinical expression of this neuronal damage, the neurological deficit, is close related to the PTE. In our studies there is an irregular evolution of the seizure incidence. After an initial phase of marked incidence, the evolution had increased a little just after the 6th month post trauma. This could be related to an association of factors: general trauma factors and neurological damage during the first days after trauma and the neuronal later reorganization. In our study the functional brain damage begins to be established by the 6th month after trauma but a relative high percentage of disturbance appears later (this is better expressed in our EEG studies). This delayed neuronal dysfunction will be of the highest importance for later seizure evolution and seizure incidence.

The second point open to discussion is the relation between the type of lesion and PTE. Although it seems evident in our studies that there is a strong relationship between the neurological lesion – expressed as neurological deficit – and PTE, it seems that the functional brain damage (general dysfunction) is by itself an important factor on PTE. This is documented by the highest incidence of PTE in the worst GCS cases and by the highest incidence of PTE in patients with general cerebral dysfunction. In our studies general cerebral and hemispheric contusions are frequent types of trauma, and frequently combined, initially, to focal lesions. These lesions determine high cerebral dysfunction and they are of the grea-test importance for the development of PTE. These findings, obtained in civilian accidents in which closed head injuries are the most common type of trauma, are different from those relating PTE to focal lesions, namely PHI, that are common in war injuries. However in such studies the PHI as other lesions were followed by great loss of cerebral tissue implying global or partial brain dysfunction. And this brain dysfunction was refered to as the most frequent symptom associated with PTE[14]. Thus it is interesting to note that the association of factors such as cerebral dysfunction and established focal neurological deficits is a combination increasing strongly the probability of existing PTE. The importance of this cerebral dysfunction will also explain the incidence of seizures and their types in relation age to groups. The disturbing of the neuronal networks (more pronounced in the worst injuries, in children or in aged people) generating abnormal potentials and giving rise to excitation of damaged structures may be responsible for the highest incidence of partial seizures.

The electroencephalographic studies here carried out open the last point for discussion. These studies documented the relevance of the evolution of the cerebral lesions on the changing patterns of the EEGs and the evolution of PTE. In spite of the early assessment of focal abnormalities on EEGs, explaining the early incidence of Psz, the changing of the EEG pattern is very high (55%) by the end of the first year after trauma. This EEG pattern is more related to the reorganization of the neurological structures than to the type of lesion. This is expressed by the higher frequency of paroxysmal activity in certain groups: children, aged persons and worst trauma cases. Although there are differences in their EEG expression, these groups have similar clinical evolution. The differences of EEG abnormalities may have a developmental reason. Focal EEG abnormalities are more frequent in aged persons and in worst GCS patients. Generalized abnormal EEG activity is more frequent in children, probably due to the neuronal maturation: a factor only present in children and giving rise to an increase of generalized activities in the EEG.

In conclusion, in posttraumatic epilepsy partial seizures are more frequent and of later occurrence than generalized seizures. The occurrence of seizures is related to neurological deficits and severity of brain dysfunction (which is higher in generalized or hemispheric lesions or severe temporal and partial ones). The type of seizures is related to age and trauma severity with a higher proportion of partial seizures in children and old people. Only 50% of the EEG findings at one month after trauma are stable. In patients with posttraumatic epilepsy, EEG focal abnormalities are found in more than 60% of EEG records two years after trauma. Diffuse or hemispheric lesions have a more changing EEG pattern. The percentage of normal EEGs increased in patients with GCS < 13 and the percentage of EEG focal abnormalities incresed in patients with GCS higher or equal to 13. The percentage of normal EEGs is lower in children and in old people with a relatively higher proportion of generalized activity in children and focal activity in elderly.

References

1. Caveness WF, Meirowsky AM, Rish BL, Mohr JP, Kistler JP, Dillon JO, Weiss GH (1979) The nature of posttraumatic epilepsy. J Neurosurg 50: 545–553
2. Dusser A, Navelet Y, Devictor D, Landrieu P (1989) Short and long-term prognostic value of the electroencephalogram in children with severe head injury. Electroencephalogr Clin Neurophysiol 73: 85–93
3. Feeney DM, Walker AE (1979) The prediction of posttraumatic epilepsy. A mathematical approach. Arch Neurol 36:8-12
4. Flint G (1988) Seizures and epilepsy. B J Neurosurg 2 (3):419–421
5. Goldstein M (1980) Traumatic Brain injury: a silent epidemic. Ann Neurol 27: 327
6. Jabbari B, Vengrow MI, Salazar AM, Harper MG, Smutok MA, Amin D (1986) Clinical and radiological correlate of EEG in the late phase of head injury: a study of 515 vietnam veterans. Electroenceph Clin Neurophysiol 64: 285-293.
7. Jennet B, Miller JD, Braakman R (1974) Epilepsy after non-missile depressed fracture. J Neurosurg 41: 208–216
8. Martins da Silva A, Rocha Vaz A, Ribeiro I, Melo AR, Nunes B, Correia M (1990) Controversies in Posttraumatic Epilepsy. Acta Neurochir (Wien) [Suppl] 50: 48–51
9. Omaya AK, Gemarelli TA (1987) Experimental head injury. In: Vinken P (ed) Handbook of clinical neurology, Chapt. 4, pp 67–90
10. Pagni CA (1990) Posttraumatic epilepsy. Incidence and prophylaxis. Acta Neurochir [Suppl] 50: 38–47
11. Pampiglione G (1975) Early neurophysiological assessment after insult to the central nervous system. In: Pontei R, Fitzsimons DW (eds) Outcome of severe damage to the central nervous system. Elsevier, Excerpta Medica, North Holland, pp 263–277
12. Pechadre JC, Lauxerois M, Colnet G, Commun C, Dimicoli C, Bonnard M, Gilbert J, Chabannes (1991) Prevention de l'épilepsie post-traumatique tardive par phénytoïne dans les traumatismes crâniens graves. Suivi durant 2 ans. Presse Méd 20: 841–845
13. Salazar AM, Amin D, Vance SC, Grafman JG, Schlesselman S, Bruck D (1987) Epilepsy after penetrating head injury: effects of Lesion Location. In: Wolf P, Dam M, Janz D, Dreifuss FE (eds) Advances in epileptology, Vol 16. Raven Press, New York, pp 753–757
14. Salazar AM, Grafman J, Vance SC, Weigartner H, Dillon JP, Ludlow C (1986) Consciousness and amnesia after penetrating head injury: neurology and anatomy. Neurology 36: 178–187
15. Temkim NR, Dikman SS, Wilnsky AJ, Keihm J, Chabal S, Winn RH (1990) A randomized, double-blind study of phenytoin for the prevention of post-traumatic seizures. N Engl J Med 323: 497–502
16. Walker AE (1989) Posttraumatic epilepsy in World War II veterans. Surg Neurol 32: 235–236
17. Weiss G, Caveness WF (1972) Prognostic factors in the persistence of posttraumatic epilepsy. J Neurosurg 37(2): 164–169
18. Willmore LJ, Sypert GW, Munson JB (1978) Recurrent seizures induced by cortical iron injection: a model of posttraumatic epilepsy. Ann Neurol 4: 329–336

Correspondence: Prof. Dr. A. Martins da Silva, Serviço de Neurofisiologia, Hospital de Santo António, 4000 Porto, Portugal.

Acta Neurochir (1992) [Suppl] 55: 64–67
© Springer-Verlag 1992

Risk Factors for Late Posttraumatic Epilepsy

A. De Santis, E. Sganzerla, D. Spagnoli, L. Bello, and **F. Tiberio**

Institute of Neurosurgery, University of Milan, Milano, Italy

Summary

The usually accepted risk factors for late post-traumatic seizures (LPTS) are those identified years ago by Jennet: early post-traumatic seizure (EPTS), depressed fracture, intracranial haematoma.

Prolonged unconsciousness (PTA > 24 hrs) is another factor usually added. More recently, personal experience of the Authors and the data of the literature, compel us to question the validity of known risk factors based on clinical data. Authors believe that the identification of patients at risk for LPTS depends mainly on the precise definition of trauma severity and on CT or surgically documented lesions of brain substance. Three groups of patients, characterized by the presence of one or more of the accepted risk factors of LPTS, have been studied. In our experience, while in adults the presence of documented cortico-subcortical lesions represents the main risk factor of LPTS, in children the appearance of EPTS per se increases the risk of LPTS, irrespective of the presence of documented brain lesions. Alteration of consciousness without a focal lesion, even if prolonged and severe, is not a risk factor for LPTS.

Keywords: Late posttraumatic epilepsy; risk factors.

Introduction

Risk factors for post-traumatic epilepsy (PTE) are still debated, in spite of the large number of articles published on this subject. Widely accepted risk factors of PTE are those identified by Jennet[16]: early seizure, depressed fracture, intracranial haematoma.

PTA lasting more than 24 hours is also considered as an adverse factor. Annegers[1] discussing the relations between early and late seizures stressed the need to better define the severity of traumatic cerebral lesions. The validity of this recommendation has been widely confirmed by the extensive utilization of CT scan in brain injured patients. Most authors have indeed found a correlation between the appearance of seizures and severity of brain injury. However, while the definition of the severity of the injury may be easy for some patients (i.e. those submited to surgery) the same definition may be

quite difficult for patients in which trauma severity has been defined only by clinical evaluation. Diffuse brain injury with prolonged coma, for instance, is classified as "severe" just as would be a large brain contusion in a "silent" brain area producing secondary loss of consciousness and coma. It is however unquestionable that the two patients will have a radically different probability for the development of post-traumatic seizures. The need for a better definition of the type and severity of traumatic brain lesions in civilian head injuries results also from our experience[12,13] and has been confirmed by D'Alessandro[3, 4, 5, 6].

In this report we present the cumulative data of patients studied in our department with regard to risk factors for late post-traumatic epilepsy.

Clinical Material and Methods

Early post-traumatic seizures, (as defined by Jennet[16], i.e. seizures occuring within one week from trauma).

To define the role of early seizures in relation to the appearance of late seizures we reviewed three groups of patients:

1) 4831 adult patients admitted to the Department of Neurosurgery of the University of Milano from 1971 to 1981 following head injuries of various severity. None of the patients considered was affected by epilepsy before trauma. This first group is characterized by the fact that most of the patients were not submitted to CT scan.

2) 1420 adult patients admitted during the period 1984-1989. All these patients were submitted to one or more CT scans.

3) 3302 paediatric head injured patients (2 months to 14 years) admitted to our department in the period 1965–1981. CT studies were available for only a few patients.

Impaired Consciousness

To study the relevance of this particular risk factor 60 patients (31 children and 29 adults, age ranging from 2 to 60 years), admitted in the period 1982-1987 have been studied. All these patients were characterized by immediate posttraumatic coma associated with diffuse brain injury (diffuse axonal injury and/or diffuse brain swelling). All patients have been studied with serial CT scans.

All patients survived their injury and were followed-up (follow-up 1–8 years).

Acute Intracranial Complication (Depressed Fractures, Intracranial Haematomas and Brain Contusion)

For the evaluation of this risk factor, 98 patients admitted in the period 1986–1988 have been studied. These patients have been selected from among a group of 600 consecutive head injured patients admitted to our department, according to the following criteria: CT documented focal brain lesions, submitted either to surgical or conservative treatment, intracranial extracerebral haematomas and depressed fractures, all submitted to surgery. Among 126 selected patients 98 (65 males and 33 females, aged 5–76 years) could be followed up for a sufficient time span (15–55 months, mean 28.5 months). There were 3 subdural haematomas, 18 extradural clots, 49 small brain contusions who did not require surgical treatment and 28 large focal brain contusions associated with subdural haematomas, or depressed fractures all submitted to surgery. 40 of these patients had pharmacological prophylaxis for PTE with phenobarbital.

Results

Early Seizures

In the first group of 4831 adult patients, 129 (2.7%) had early seizures. 85 of them could be discharged from hospital. 52 have been followed-up (mean follow-up 5.6 years). 17 of these patients were operated on: 14 brain contusions, 2 extradural haematomas. In one case no lesion was found at surgery. 35 patients were treated conservatively. Among the 52 followed-up patients, 12 (23%) had late posttraumatic seizures. 9 of them had been submitted to surgery; i. e. 53% of operated patients with early seizures also had late seizures. Only 3 conservatively treated patients (8.5%) with early seizures developed LPTS. In conclusion, 75% of patients with LPTS had an important focal brain lesion that needed surgical treatment.

In the second group of 1420 adults, 41 (2.9%) had EPTS. Of these, 5 died from the severity of their brain injury. 32 of the 36 discharged patients could be followed-up (1–4 years). 3 of them (9.4%) developed LPTS. All of them had a CT documented focal brain lesion. Also for this group the presence of documented brain lesions seems to be the main risk factor for LPTS, irrespective of EPTS.

Among the group of 3302 children, 165 (5%) EPTS were observed. 85 of them have been followed-up from 1 to 14 years (average 5 years). 20 (23%) of them had LPTS. At variance with adults, only 40% of LPTS were associated with a documented focal brain lesion, while in as much as 60% of children with EPTS followed by LPTS, no sure brain lesion was noted and in many of them the head injury had been trivial.

Impaired Consciousness

In the group of severely head injured patients with diffuse brain lesions (diffuse axonal injury or diffuse brain swelling) and prolonged coma (GCS 4 = 14: GCS 5 = 25; GCS 6 = 13; GCS 7 = 8 on admission) only one patient had a single early seizure, while no patient had LPTS. Severe alteration of consciousness per se seems therefore not predictive of LPTS.

Acute Intracranial Complications

In the group of 98 patients with CT documented focal intracranial lesions, 12 had LPTS (12.2%). According to the type of brain lesion, 8 pts had large focal brain contusion-haematomas, 3 had small contusions and 1 demonstrated an extradural blood collection. Thus 91.6% of pts with LPTS had a CT documented focal brain lesion. Seizures nevertheless, developed in 28% of patients with large brain contusions submitted to surgery, and only in 6% of patients with small brain lesions treated conservatively and in 4.7% of cases with pure extracerebral collections.

Discussion

On the basis of the results of this clinical investigation on a large number of head injured patients, who were selected for the presence of one or more of the commonly recognized risk factors for LPTS, the following remarks can be made.

The relevance of EPTS appears to be different in children than in adults and details have been decribed in previous papers[8, 9].

In our series the prevalence of LPTS has been particulary high among children presenting EPTS. Our figures are even higher than those reported by Jennet[16], Hendrik and Harris[15] and Stöwesand and Bues[17] who all are of the opinion that EPTS increase the risk of LPTS. LPTS have appeared in all types of head traumas, but, as expected, have been even higher in operated children. Also when EPTS had a seemingly "functional" origin, the percentage of LPTS has been much higher than that observed in series without EPTS[10]. In agreement with most authors we therefore confirm the opinion that the observation of EPTS in children increases the risk of LPTS.

Although the prevalence of LPTS among adults with EPTS is seemingly high[1, 2, 14, 16, 18, 19], the majority of our patients was also harbouring a focal brain lesion. As a matter of fact, 75% of LPTS were observed among patients submitted to surgery for traumatic intracranial complications. Moreover the prevalence of LPTS (23%) has been similar to that observed among patients without EPTS but with comparable severity and type of intracranial lesions[7, 11, 13]. The impression that the type of brain lesion more than the occurence EPTS determines an increased risk of LPTS seems to be confirmed by our smaller group of patients with EPTS who all have been submitted to CT and in whom the type and severity of anatomical brain disruption has been ascertained.

In conclusion we do believe that in adults EPTS are not a risk factor for LPTS per se but increase the risk of LPTS only if associated with documented focal brain lesions. Annegers[1] reaches similar conclusions in his study on adult and peadiatric patients in which he finds a correlation between EPTS and LPTS only in some groups of adults and writes that "this association might disappear if severity were defined more precisely". Also D'Alessandro[3, 4, 5, 6] believes that the only risk factors are CT documented brain lesions while clinical factors like EPTS or PTA have not to be considered as such.

The belief of most authors that clinical factors like PTA should be considered relevant in the prediction of LPTS seems to be completely denied by our series of patients selected for the presence of severe and prolonged alterations of consciousness without focal brain lesions. The overestimation of PTA and/or coma as risk factor for LPTS might have been due to the fact that it was considered as evidence of the severity of the brain lesion and possibly of widespread cortical damage. As we all have learned that prolonged traumatic coma may occur also in the absence of relevant cortical lesions (diffuse white matter damage) we may also understand why severe alterations of consciousness may not be related to LPTS. This opinion was already reported by Hendrik and Harris[15] who wrote that at variance with the common opinions "Walker maintains that loss of consciousness is brainstem dysfunction and is not associated with epilepsy".

That the presence of a documented focal brain lesion (cortico-subcortical brain disruptions) is the main risk factor for the development of LPTS has again been shown by our group of patients selected for the presence of intracranial post-traumatic complications. Already in 1935 Symons[18] stressed that "in the great majority of cases, the cause of traumatic epilepsy is direct injury to the brain substance". The main problem in determining the individual risk of LPTS is the precise neuroradiological diagnosis of the type of intracranial lesion also in patients with minimal posttraumatic brain dysfunction. In our experience other factors like the dimension of the brain lesion (lower incidence of LPTS in small lesions)

and the coexistence of alchool abuse should be taken into account.

Conclusions

The generally accepted risk factors for LPTS are: EPTS, depressed fractures, intracranial haematomas, PTA. According to our results EPTS should not be considered as a risk factor for LPTS in adults while it seems to increase their risk in children. Prolonged unconsciousness without focal brain damage should not be considered a risk factor for LPTS. Focal brain lesions are the main risk factor to be considered in predicting LPTS.

References

1. Annegers JF, Grabow JD, Groover RV, Lawes ER Jr, Elveback LR, Kurland LT (1980) Seizures after head trauma: a population study. Neurology 30: 683–689
2. Caveness WF, Meirowsky AM, Rish BL, Mohr JP, Kistler JP, Dillon JD, Weiss GH (1979) The nature of pottraumatic epilepsy. J Neurosurg 50: 545–553
3. D'Alessandro R, Tinuper P, Ferrara R (1982) Confronto fra i fattori clinici e TAC nel calcolo del rischio dell'epilepsia posttraumatica. Boll Leg It Epil 39: 69–70
4. D'Alessandro R, Tinuper P, Ferrara R, Cortelli P, Pazzaglia P, Sabattini L, Frank G, Lugaresi E (1982) CT scan prediction of late post-traumatic epilepsy. J Neurol Neurosurg Psychiatry 45: 1153–1155
5. D'Alessandro R, Ferrara R, Cortelli P, Tinuper P, Pazzaglia P, Lugaresi E (1983) Post traumatic eplilepsy prediction and prophylaxis: open problems. Arch Neurol 40: 831 Letter
6. D'Alessandro R, Ferrara R, Benassi G, Lenzi PG, Sabattini L (1988) Computed tomographic scans in posttraumatic epilepsy. Arch Neurol 45: 42–43
7. De Santis A, Ravagnati L, Sironi V, Ettorre G (1982) Controllo EEG seriato e clinico di 100 severi traumatizzati cranici in età adulta. Riv It EEG Neurofisiol Clin 5: 99–100
8. De Santis A, Granata G, Ravagnati L, Rampini P, Sina C, Caprici E (1983) Head injury and early epileptic seizures in adults. Advances in Neurotraumatology, Excerpta Medica. International Congress Series 612: 313–315
9. De Santis A, Rampini P, Ravagnati L, Sina C, Granata G, Capricci E, Vaccari U (1983) Early epilepsy in 165 juvenile head injured patients. Advances in neurotraumatology, Excerpta Medica. International Congress Series 612: 310–313
10. De Santis A, Rampini P, Granata G (1983) Epilessia posttraumatica in età infantile: controllo su una serie di traumatizzati cranici in 6 anni consecutivi. Riv It EEG Neurofisiol Clin [Suppl] 1: 285–286
11. De Santis A, Rampini P, Granata G (1983) Epilessia posttraumatica in età adulta: controllo su una serie di traumatizzati cranici in 6 anni consecutivi. Riv It EEG Neurofisiol Clin Suppl 1: 287–288
12. De Santis A, Rampini P, Sganzerla EP, Guerra P, Tiberio F, Ducati A (1988) Coma cerebrale traumatico in assenza di lesioni focali ed insorgenza di epilessia. Boll Lega It Epil 62/63: 79–82

13. De Santis A, Spagnoli D, Resta F, Sganzerla E (1990) Profilassi antiepilettica e trauma cranio-cerebrale. Boll Lega It Epil 70/71: 363–365

14. Evans JH (1963) The significance of early post traumatic epilepsy. Neurology 207–212

15. Hendrick EB, Harris L (1968) Post traumatic epilepsy in children. J Trauma 8: 547–556

16. Jennet B (1975) Epilepsy after non-missile head injury, 2nd Ed. Heinemann, London

17. Stöwesand D, Bues E (1970) Frühanfälle und ihre Verläufe nach Hirntraumen in Kindesalter. Z Neurol 198: 201–211

18. Symons CP, Oxon MD, Lond FRCP (1935) Traumatic epilepsy. Lancet 30: 1217–1220

19. Whitty CW M (1947) Early traumatic epilepsy. Brain 70: 416-439

Correspondence and Reprints: Prof. A. De Santis, Clinica Neurochirurgica, Università di Milano, Via F. Sforza, 35, 20122 Milano, Italy.

Acta Neurochir (1992) [Suppl] 55: 68–71
© Springer-Verlag 1992

Mental Deterioration at Epilepsy Onset: A Hypothesis

H. Meinardi[1], **A.P. Aldenkamp**[1], and **B. Nunes**[2]

[1] Instituut voor Epilepsiebestrijding, Heemstede, The Netherlands, [2] Serviço de Neurofisiologia-Hospital Geral de Santo Antonio, Porto, Portugal

Summary

In this study, we hypothesized a type of mental deterioration in epilepsy, characterized as a discontinued, cascading process, i. e. a sudden mental decline in a limited time interval, immediately after the onset of the seizures. The posttraumatic epilepsy model (PTE) may appear to be exceptionally useful in avoiding one of the major methodological obstacles for testing this hypotesis, i. e. the unavailability of test results obtained with the same battery of tests prior to and directly after the onset of the seizures. We propose a multicentre study in which a large group of patients are assessed, after recovering from the direct aftermath of head injury, but before the onset of PTE. This baseline provides an opportunity for longitudinal follow-up. Full recovery from head injury before the onset of PTE is to be expected in the mild and moderate groups of closed head injury patients. In this category, approximately 2000 head injured patients have to be assessed to obtain a resonable group of approximately 100–200 PTE patients.

This group will be followed during the critical period of 2–3 years after the onset of epilepsy.

Keywords: Epilepsy; deterioration; posttraumatic epilepsy; seizures.

Introduction

The notion of mental deterioration in epilepsy is of great concern to parents of children when a first diagnosis of epilepsy is made and also, but obviously in a different context, for adults with late onset of epilepsy. Whether or not the fear is realistic that epilepsy will cause mental deterioration remains a matter of debate.

Patients, treated in our epilepsy centre suffer from treatment resistant epilepsies, and are mostly referred several years after the onset. Therefore progressive deterioration as a function of the seizures or other epileptic factors should be noticed in our centre.

Despite three types of studies: one in children[1], one in adults, using long-term follow up of neurological and clinical parameters[20], and one in the mentally handi-capped with epilepsy[10], we could not confirm the hypothesized deterioration in these patients.

This is in line with several other studies such as the retrospective study of Rodin *et al.* (1986), Bourgeois *et al.* (1983), Seidenberg *et al.* (1981), Dodrill (1986).

Method

We used the technique of metanalysis[13], combining the results of several studies to generate new hypotheses.

This analysis revealed, that the lenght of the period between age of onset of epilepsy and the first assessment possibly forms an important intervening factor. In the aforementioned study by Aldenkamp, most of the children, had an age of onset several years before the first assessment was carried out (ranging from 4.2 years to 11.7 years). Consequently, a potentially deteriorating effect of the epilepsy could have *preceded* the assessments. In accordance with these findings, the Full-scale IQ-scores in the first assessment in this study were already on a subnormal level (Full-Scale IQ: 84.7), despite normal school achievement in the past.

We therefore hypothesize that the onset of epilepsy entails a reset of brain function, within a relatively short period (i. e. 2–3 years), which will stabilize after a while. The absence of significant IQ-loss during follow-up would merely demonstrate the stable phase, following the actual period of deterioration. This would be in line with the negative findings in the previously mentioned studies, that were carried out several years after the epilepsy onset, whereas the critical period with mental decline might be the first years after the onset.

This hypothesis proposed that our current model for deterioration needs further consideration. This deterioration may not necessarily be characterized by a continuous process as illustrated in Fig. 1. Figure 2 illustrates the hypothesized model in which deterioration is a step-like process, i. e. sudden and limited in time, directly after the onset of the seizures. This hypothesis is supported by the study by Rodin *et al.* (1986). In this study, convincing evidence for deterioration could not be found, although intelligence was generally on a subnormal level (FS.IQ: 87 at the re-test for the non-remitting patients) and mental arrest without loss of abilities was obtained. Follow-up started several years after the onset of the epilepsy and could well be within the hypothesized stable phase, following deterioration. Most prospective studies also start the follow-up period several years after the age of onset[9, 23].

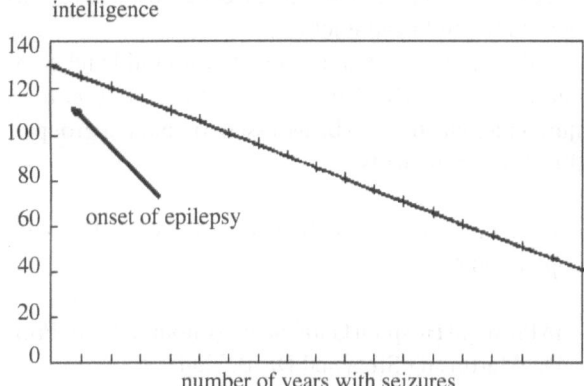

Fig. 1. Deterioration as a continuous process

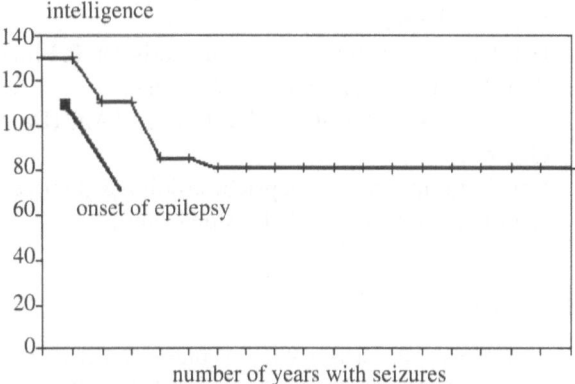

Fig. 2. Deterioration as a step-like process

Alpherts analyzed cognitive performance for children in different age-groups from seven up to eighteen years[2]. The results show, that performance levels in younger age groups are about the same for children with epilepsy and normal controls. Differences between the epilepsy group and controls emerge in a relatively short period, followed by stabilization, resulting in more or less parallel curves with performance in the epilepsy group at subnormal level. This pattern can be explained by normal age effects: tasks have more differentiating power after the age of 10 years and are therefore more sensitive for detecting genuine function disorders. An alternative explanation may be the aforementioned step-like deterioration, directly after the onset of the seizures followed by a stable phase at subnormal level. The two figures (Figs. 3 and 4), mentioned by Alpherts is his study may be in accordance with this explanation[2].

Discussion

To test this hypothesis would require the analysis of cognitive function in people before and after the onset of the epilepsy, preferably with the same methods. As patients may have unrecognized or untreated seizures, the actual follow-up could not start after the 'official' diagno-sis of epilepsy. In the study by Bourgeois and coworkers, unrecognized seizures were found in a significant part of the study group[4]. Moreover in most patients anti-epileptic treatment is started immediately after the onset of the seizures, complicating the study of mental functioning. Most types of drug treatment also have a serious impact on cognition[24].

A more satisfactory answer to the topic of deterioration can be found, when we apply the post-traumatic epilepsy (PTE) model[19], that appears to be exceptionally useful in avoiding one of the major methodological obstacles, i. e. the unavailability of test results obtained with the same battery of tests prior to and directly after the onset of the seizures. If we are able to assess a large group of patients, after recovering from the direct aftermath of head injury, but before the onset of PTE, we may have a baseline for longitudinal follow-up during the initial phase after the onset of the epilepsy and during the following years.

In fact the use of the post-traumatic epilepsy model has already been applied to study the effects of epilepsy in the "Vietnam Head Injury Study"[22], patients in with penetrating head injures (PHI) and severe focal brain damage. Full recovery after the acute phase is not possible here. Consequently deterioration was in particular associated with the amount of loss of brain tissue in these patients.

In closed-head injury (CHI) patients a distinction has to be made between the acute, subacute and chronic effects of head injury. The acute effects can be alarming, such as gross retrograde amnesia, accelerated forgetting and disorientated behaviour. During the subacute phase, patients report slower thinking and difficulties in doing two things simultaneously. They also report themselves as irritable and oversensitive to stimulation such as noise or flashing lights. The reports about the concentration and 'slowing' disorders appear to be related to severity of injury[27]. Both complaints have been confirmed with neuropsychological tasks, in acute stages and within months after injury. CHI patients need more time for information processing and have difficulties in divided attention tasks[26]. Van Zomeren and Deelman (1978), evaluating chronic effects with a choice reaction-time test, observed no differences between a mild injured group and normal healthy controls, and found full recovery for a moderately injured group after about half a year. Only for the severe group were persistent effects found during the total follow-up period. These chronic effects after severe head injury may be restricted to slow information processing[6]. In a group with severe CHI and intracranial haematomas Mandleberg and Brooks (1975) obtained full recovery of WAIS IQ-scores after one year follow-up. This recovery was more gradual for the performance subtests, possibly because of the greater impact of speed factors on these tests.

Type of Assessment

It follows from the criteria mentioned above that, in our proposed study, the first baseline measurement has to be assessed at approximately three to six months after the head injury. A second criterion is the type of head injury. If PHI-patients and patients with severe CHI are excluded, this baseline will measure cognitive function and intelligence level after recovery from the trauma and prior to the onset of epilepsy.

The criteria for defining recovery are: early assessment of the posttraumatic amnesia (PTA), orientation, behaviour and mood, using the Glascow Coma Scale and the Galveston Orientation and Amnesia Test (GOAT) and the Neurobehavioural Rating Scale[12, 3, 17]. Lenght of coma, scores on the GCS and lenght of PTA have prognostic value and indicate the severity of injury and the probability of permanent cognitive defects of the injury itself[5]. A head injury is considered as mild with GCS scores ranging form 13 to 15 and moderate with scores 9-12[3]. When PTA is lenghty (more than 3 months) these scores may underestimate the actual cognitive impairment. In addition, as early as possible simple cognitive tasks, such as reaction-time tasks (when possible supplemented with the registration of event-related potentials) and screening for amnesia and aphasia, may add an indication of initial cognitive deficit. Extensive neuropsychological assessment can proceed when 85% accuracy on the GOAT is achieved. Levin and coworkers show that particular attention is needed for the phenomenon of impaired acquisition and accelerated forgetting, possibly related to the vulnerability of the temporal lobes for the diffuse effects of CHI[16]. This may be caused by the tendency for damage to occur in centripetal progression, with the outermost structures most likely to be affected[3].

A Multicentre Study to Test the Deterioration Hypothesis

The incidence of mild forms of head injury is estimated for the USA at 610,000 cases within one year[7]. A smaller estimate is 325,000 annual hospital admissions with more than seventy percent classified as mild[14].

The incidence of posttraumatic epilepsy (PTE) is between 2,5% (mild CHI) to 50% (in PHI; Salazar *et al.*, 1987). Approximately 50% of the patients, who develop epilepsy, do so within a period of 12 months after the head trauma (Hauser and Hesdorffer, 1990). An increased incidence of PTE is reported to occur with severe as opposed to mild head injuries[11].

In this study we include patients with mild and moderate forms of CHI, therefore an estimated 2000 head injured patients have to be assessed to obtain a group of 100–200 PTE patients.

To achieve this, a multicentre trial will start with cooperation of:

– In Portugal Hospital Geral Santo António, Porto (Prof. Dr. Martins da Silva and Dr. B. Nunes).
– In Germany Charlottenburg/Freie Universität Berlin (Dr. H. J. Meencke).
– In the UK, The National Hospital/Chalfont Centre (Dr. S. Shorvon and Dr. P. Thompson).
– In the Netherlands:
   Het Radboudziekenhuis (Prof. Dr. Goris, Dr. P. Eling, Prof. Dr. H. Meinardi and Dr. W. Renier).
   The University Hospital of Amsterdam, AMC (Dr. J. Overweg).
   Het Instituut voor Epilepsiebestrijding/Rijkuniversiteit Leiden (Prof. Dr. A. P. Aldenkamp).

References

1. Aldenkamp AP, Alpherts WCJ, De Bruïne D, Dekker MJA (1990) Test-retest variability in children with epilepsy – a comparison of WISC-R subtest profiles. Epilepsy Res 7: 165–172
2. Alpherts WCJ, Aldenkamp AP (1990) Computerized neuropsychological assessment of cognitive functioning in children with epilepsy. In: Aldenkamp AP, Dodson WE (eds) Epilepsy and education. Cognitive factors in learning behavior. Epilepsia [Suppl] 4: S 35–S40
3. Binder LM, Rattok J (1989) Assessment of postconcussive syndrome after mild head injury. In: Lezak M (ed) Assessment of the behavioral consequences of head trauma. Allan R. Liss Publ, New York, pp 37–48
4. Bourgeois BFD, Presky AL, Palkes HS, Talent BK, Busch SG (1983) Intelligence in epilepsy: a prospective study in children. Ann Neurol 14: 438–444
5. Brooks N (1989) Closed head trauma: assessing the common cognitive problems. In: M. Lezak (ed) Assessment of the behavioral consequences of head trauma. R. Liss Publ, New York, pp 61–85
6. Brouwer WH, Ponds RWHM, Wolffelaar van PC, Zomeren van AH (1989) Divided attention 5 to 10 years after severe closed head injury. Cortex 25: 219–230
7. Caveness WF (1977) Incidence of craniocerebral trauma in the United States, 1970–1975. Ann Neurol 1: 507
8. Caveness WF (1978) Epilepsy, a product of trauma in our time. Epilepsia 19: 177–183
9. Dodrill CB (1986) Correlates of generalized tonic-clonic seizures with intellectual, neuropsychological, emotional and social function in patients with epilepsy. Epilepsia 27: 399–411

10. Forceville EJM, Aldenkamp AP, Alpherts WCJ, Dekker MJA, Schelvis, AJ (1992) Subtest profiles of the Wisc-R and WAIS in mentally retarded patients with epilepsy. J Ment Def Res 36: 124-145

11. Jennet WB (1969) Epilepsy after blunt (nonmissile) head injuries. In: Walker AE, Caveness WF, CritchleyM (eds) The late effects of head injury, pp 201–214. Charles C Thomas, Springfield III

12. Kampen DL, Grafman J (1989) Neuropsychological evaluation of penetrating head injury. In: Lezak M (ed) Assessment of the behavioral consequences of head trauma. Allan R Liss Publ, New York, pp 49–60

13. Kerlinger FN (1973) Foundations of behavioral research. Holt, Rinheart and Winston, London

14. Kraus JF, Black MA, Hesson N (1984) The incidence of acute brain injury and serious impairment in a defined population. Am J Epidemiol 119:186–201

15. Lesser RP, Lüders H, Wyllie E, Dinner DS, Morris HH (1986) Mental deterioration in epilepsy. Epilepsia 27 [Suppl 2]: S 105–123

16. Levin HS, High WM, Eisenberg HM (1988) Learning and forgetting during posttraumatic amnesia in head injured patients. J Neurol Neurosurg Psychiatry 51: 14–20

17. Lezak M (1989) Assessment of the behavioral consequences of head trauma. Allan R Liss Publ, New York

18. Mandleberg IA, Brooks DN (1975) Cognitive recovery after severe head injury. J Neurol Neurosurg Psychiatry 38: 1121–1126

19. Martins da Silva A, Rocha Vaz A, Nunes B, Correia M, Ribeiro I, Melo AR, Mendonça D (1989) Factors associated with Post traumatic epilepsy. Abstract presented at the 18th IEC, New Delhi

20. Meinardi H, Beun AM, Aldenkamp AP, Nunes B, Engelsman M, Forceville E (1990) Mental deterioration in a population with intractable epilepsy. In: Pisani F, Perucca G, Avanzini F, Richens A (eds) New antiepileptic drug. Epilepsy Res [Suppl] 3: 7–13

21. Rodin EA, Schmaltz S, Twitty G (1986) Intellectual functions of patients with childhood-onset epilepsy. Dev Med Child Neurol 28: 25–33

22. Salazar AM, Grafman J, Jabbari B, Vance SC, Amin D (1987) Epilepsy and cognitive loss after penetrating head injury. In: Wolf P, Dam M, Dreifuss FE (eds) Advances in epileptology, Vol 16. Raven Press, New York, pp 627–631

23. Seidenberg M, O'Leary DS, Giordani B, Berent S, Boll TJ (1981) Test-retest changes of epilepsy patients: assessing the influence of practice effects. J Clin Neuropsychol 3: 237–255

24. Trimble (1990) Antiepileptic drugs, cognitive function and behavior in children; evidence from recent studies. In: Aldenkamp AP, Dodson WE (eds) Epilepsy and education. Cognitive factors in learning behavior. Epilepsia [Suppl] 4: S 30–S34

25. Zomeren AH van, Deelman G (1978) Long-term recovery of visual reaction time after closed head injury. J Neurol Neurosurg Psychiatry 4: 452–457

26. Zomeren AH van, Brouwer WH, Deelman BG (1984) Attentional deficits: the riddles of selectivity, speed and alerteness. In: DN Brooks (ed) Closed head injury. Oxford University Press, pp 74–107

27. Zomeren AH van, Burg W van den (1985) Residual complaints of patients two years after severe head injury. J Neurol Neurosurg Psychiatry 48: 21–28

Correspondence: Prof. Dr. H. Meinardi, Instituut voor Epilepsiebestrijding, Achterweg 5, 2103 SW Heemstede, The Netherlands.

Acta Neurochir (1992) [Suppl] 55: 72–74

Rehabilitation After Severe Head Injury

R. A. Frowein, D. Terhaag, K. auf der Haar, K.-E. Richard, and **R. Firsching**

Neurosurgical Department of the University of Cologne, Köln, Federal Republic of Germany

Summary

123 survivors of severely head injured patients presenting with coma grade III show a decreasing mean duration of coma with increasing age.

The numbers and frequency of good recovery decrease, whereas poor recovery increases with age.

Increase of the duration of coma grade III produces an increase of the mean latency and time of recovery and of the frequency of poor recovery, regardless of the age of the patients.

Increasing age does not increase the mean latency and time of recovery systematically.

The important conclusion of this analysis is, that the clinical feature of coma grade III, corresponding to GCS score of 4 and RLS of 6 and 7, indicates a different kind of brain damage at various age groups. It represents a lesser degree of brain damage for younger patients under 20, than for those over 20.

In our opinion our observations do not demonstrate a better capacity of recovery of the young patients: but the young patients show a more severe clinical picture than the older patients do, if only the clinical syndrome of coma grade III with extensor rigidity, is considered as a yardstick for comparison.

Keywords: Coma scales; rehabilitation; recovery; head trauma.

Material

Between 1974 and 1988 there were 3.384 patients with head injuries treated at our Department of Neurosurgery. 10% of these, 355 comatose patients, exhibited flexor and/or extensor-rigidity, reaching a GCS score of 4, which is equivalent to a Reaction Level Scale (RLS 85) of 6 and 7, and to a Brussel's Coma Scale (BCS) grade III[1, 3, 8, 9, 10]. The high mortality of 56% is proof of the severity of the underlying brain damage.

Among 155 survivors a close follow up in 123 patients was possible. There were 10 to 44 patients per year.

Follow up ranged from 16 years for patients injured in 1974, to 2 years for those injured in 1988. We have collected 75% of the maximal follow up time.

Distribution of Age

As in other statistics concerning patients who show coma grade III in the first days after injury, three quarters of our comatose patients were young, 6 to 25 years of age. Their age groups are the largest with 24, 27 and 19 patients in each.

Relation of Duration of Coma Grade III to Age

In the following analysis only survivors of coma grade III of one or more days duration will be considered.

Figure 1 summarizes our observations and shows that with increasing age there is a decreasing mean duration of coma grade III from 6.8 to 4.7 days.

This tendency is less evident in the mean total duration of coma, ranging between 6.9 to 9.1 days, even if extremes of more than 20 days of coma are excluded.

Illustrative Case Report

An example of the follow up of one of our patients (Rolf L., 234/74) gives our definitions:

In 1974 this six year old boy was struck by a car and was comatose immediately. He presented with extensor

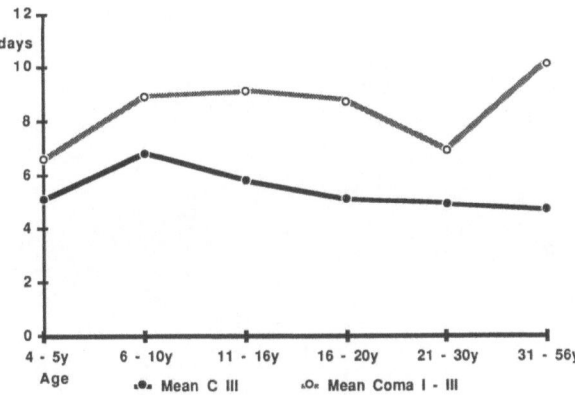

Fig. 1. Mean duration of coma grade III (Mean C III) and of all coma grades I to III (Mean Coma I–III) in relation to age

rigidity, GCS of 4, that is BCS grade III, for 4 days; paraplegia resolved after 4 months.

It took one year until he was able to attend school and to get good marks. We call this period from injury until the first definite progress the *latency of recovery*.

But at the age of 10 the boy showed retardation, manual tremor and his performance at school deteriorated.

Finally it took 7 years until he was considered to have recovered completely. We call this period until the definite recovery the *time of recovery*.

Then the young boy was able to attend a technical college, and this year, 16 years after injury, at the age of 22, he succeded in becoming a certified engineer.

Follow up Age Groups

In this manner we collected data from 123 patients on the degree of recovery, classified according to the GOS[6] as poor recovery, or severe or moderate disability, or good recovery, for each patient in relation to the intervals of 3, 6, 9 months, 1, 2, 3 and so on years after injury.

For most patients the two periods of *latency* of recovery and *time* of recovery may be clearly distinguished.

In the age group of 4–5 years old at injury 4 out of 7 patients achieved good recovery: 3 of them during a period of 1 to 2 years, in one case of 7 years. One girl remained moderately, two boys remained severely disabled after 6, 7 respectively 10 days of coma grade III. No one remained at the level of poor recovery.

The group of 24 children aged 6 to 10 years at injury have the best results: there were 10 children, that is 42% of this age group of survivors, who achieved good results.

7 patients, that is 29%, remained moderately disabled, 12% severely disabled, and another 17% did not recover at all after 3 to 26 days of coma grade III.

In this group is also the highest number of 8/24, 33% delayed recoveries after 3 and more years: 5 to good, 3 to moderate disability.

In the largest group of 27 young patients 11 to 16 years old at the time of injury, the proportion of ultimately good recovery is 27%, of moderate disability is 35%, of severe disability 27% and of poor or no recovery it is 15%.

The group of 24 patients 17 to 20 years old shows 33% good recovery and 25% of moderate disability. The recovery time was mostly 1 to 2 years. 6 out of the 24 patients, 25%, recovered later after 3 to 7 years.

By contrast, among the 23 injured patients between 21 to 30 year old, good recovery amounted only to 17%, but severe disability to 30%. Poor recovery was observed in

more than one third of these cases, 39%. One patient died 8 years after injury.

Out of 5 delayed recoveries only 1 patient achieved good results.

Among the 18 patients 31 years and older at injury only 16% good results were achieved. Only one patient, 6%, later recovered to moderate disability. One lady may overrate her assessment of a good recovery after 11 years. Half of the patients remained at the level of poor recovery.

Follow up Results

Figure 2 summarizes these follow up observations of the different age groups. Patients 6 to 10 years of age have the highest number of good recoveries; the frequency amounts to 42%.

There is a decreasing number and a decreasing frequency of good recovery from the age of 10 years on and an increasing number and frequency of poor results from

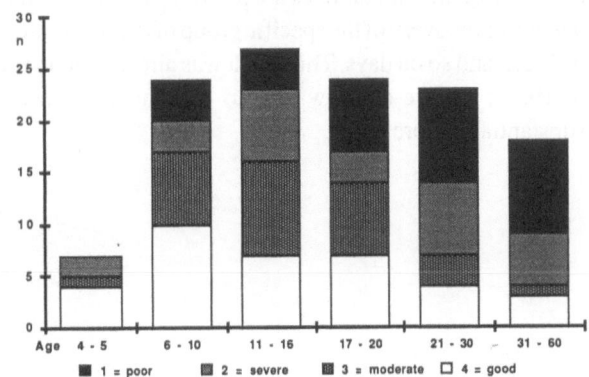

Fig. 2. Final grade of recovery after coma grade III in different age groups

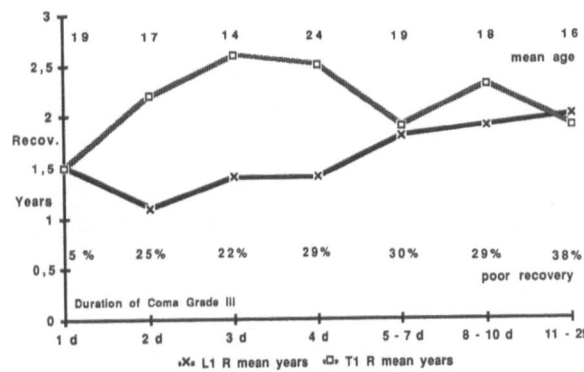

Fig. 3. Mean latency of recovery (L1R) and mean time of recovery (T1R) (in years) after coma grade III of variable duration (in days)

an age of 4 years at injury onwards. This correlation is already well known[2, 4, 7].

Latency and Time of Recovery in Relation to Coma Duration

But the correlation between the duration of coma and the periods of recovery is less well established.

Therefore we have examined groups of patients with the same duration of coma grade III for 1, 2, 3 and so on days, and we have calculated the mean values of the latency and of the time of recovery for the variable duration of coma grade III (Fig. 3). One of the results is, that increasing duration of coma grade III produces a slight increase of the mean latency of recovery (L 1 R) ranging from 1 to 2 years. The increase of the mean time of recovery from 1.5 to 2.5 years is less constant.

With coma grade III of 3 days duration occurs the longest mean time of recovery of 2.6 years; but there is also the lowest mean age of 14 years.

These figures do not include the additional increasing part of 25% to 38% of poor results with no recovery at all.

The second result of this analysis is, that increasing mean age of the patients does not prolong, on average, the latency of recovery of the specific group of coma duration of 1, 2, 3 and so on days. This result was already recorded in 1987[5]; but we are now able to demonstrate it with substantially more cases.

References

1. Brihaye J, Frowein RA, Lindgren S, Loew F, Stroobrandt G (1978) Report on the Meeting of the W.F.N.S. Neuro-Traumatology Commitee, Brussels 19–23 Sept. 1976. I, Coma Scaling. Acta Neurochir (Wien) 40: 181–186
2. Brooks N (1984) Closed head injury. Oxford University Press, New York Toronto
3. Frowein RA (1976) Classification of coma. Acta Neurochir (Wien) 34: 5–10
4. Frowein RA, Haar K auf der, Terhaag D (1980) Assessment of coma, rebility of prognosis. Neurosurg Rev 3: 67–74
5. Frowein RA, Firsching R (1988) Personality after head injury. Acta Neurochir (Wien) [Suppl] 44: 70–73
6. Jennett WB, Bond MR (1975) Assessment of outcome after severe brain damage. Lancet 1: 480–484
7. Richard KE, Frowein RA, Hashimoto T (1982) Prognose traumatischer Mittelhirnsyndrome bei Kindern und Jugendlichen. In: Müller N (ed) Das traumatische Mittelhirnsyndrom und die Rehabilitation schwerer Schädelhirntraumen. Springer, Berlin Heidelberg New York, pp 23–30
8. Stalhammar D, Starmark J-E (1986) Assessment of responsiveness in head injury patients. In: Lindgren S (ed) Modern concepts of neurotraumatology. Acta Neurochir (Wien) [Suppl] 36: 91–94
9. Starmark J-E (1988) Analysis "coma scales". Thesis, Göteborg 1988, ISBN 91-7900-424-5
10. Teasdale G, Jennett B (1974) Assessment of coma and impaired consciousness. Lancet II: 81–84

Correspondence: Prof. Dr. R. A. Frowein, Geibel Strasse 22, D-W-5000 Köln 41, Federal Republic of Germany.

Acta Neurochir (1992) [Suppl] 55: 75–79
© Springer-Verlag 1992

Social-Economic Impact of Head Injury

J. Haase

Department of Neurosurgery, Aalborg Hospital, Aalborg, Denmark

Summary

The socio-economic costs of traffic road accidents were analysed data epidemiological studies and compared with reported data. The costs are calculated as a function of accident type and vehicle involved, severity of head trauma, patients individual characteristics, type of care – intensive and emergency services, other hospital bed costs, including recovering and rehabilitation such as in-and out-patient services. Finally the costs of repairing materials (cars, walls, roads, etc.) are also estimated. The author concludes that the medical doctor must take part in compiling the statistics so as to be able to discuss the economics of injury and the social priorities.

Keywords: Social impact; medical economics; recovery; head trauma; traffic accidents.

Introduction

The WHO has suggested that at the latest by 2000 A.C. the number of deaths due to accidents shall be reduced by at least 25%. For that reason the number of traffic deaths must be reduced to less than 20 per 100.000 inhabitants or for countries that are already under this to less than 15 per 100.000. As all of the European countries have accepted the WHO-suggestion, we neurosurgeons need to have a know-ledge of statistics and economical theories related to traffic accidents as advisers for our administrators and politicians[2]. Within the hospitals we have excellent statistics such as the costs of hospital bed days[3, 5]. We know exactly how many hospital bed days are used for victims of traffic accidents. From the Danish statistics a patient, who dies from a traffic accident, is estimated to stay in the hospital a mean of 6 days[5]. Among those involved in major traffic accidents, not related to death, the male stays a mean of 8,7 days and the females a mean of 17,0 days in the hospital (Table 1).

With an apparently sufficient registration of major injuries and deaths administrations simply multiply these figures by the cost of a hospital day to get an estimate of the costs related to traffic accidents – an estimate that is being used for budget discussions.

These budgets include technological inventions and with the increase of money spend on hospital well-fare the technological evolution is being hindered. Can we as doctors rely on our official statistics? Can we accept the hospital budgets as they are? The Odense Traffic Accident Analysing Study Group made an epidemiological study at the Island of Fyn with an accurate determination of the number of all traffic accidents. The Island of Fyn is epidemiological an excellent representative of Denmark and serves for the revised figures I have deducted for the whole country (Table 2).

As can be seen the official data on deaths and those of the Odense study are similar. However, when looking into the major injuries the Odense group found 6.272 more cases or an increase of 74% compared with that officially stated. Looking into the minor injuries the figures are even more frightening, missing 25.114 accidents or 384% more than that given by official figures. This clearly demonstrates how important it is that doctors are involved in making the statistics! No computerisation of data is better than the data fed into the computers.

Table 1. *Number of Hospital Bed Days*

Killed		6 (estimated)				
Major		male			female	
Car	8,7	SD	14,4	17,0	SD	34,7
MC	14,1	SD	21,2	10,8	SD	10,8
Bike	5,6	SD	8,6	6,8	SD	6,8
Ped	14,2	SD	21,3	23,4	SD	28,5

Table 2. *Number of Accidents in Denmark 1980*

	Car	MC	Bike	Ped.	Total	
Deaths	337	131	84	138	690	official
	337	131	84	138	*690*	revised
Major	3.638	2.148	1.465	1.204	8.455	official
	4.898	3.333	4.719	1.777	*14.727*	revised
Minor	3.591	1.339	1.068	537	6.535	official
	8.155	4.562	16.944	1.988	*31.649*	revised
Total	7.566	3.618	2.617	1.879	15.680	official
	13.390	8.026	21.747	3.903	*47.066*	revised

Italics = Revised figures.

Looking into the neurosurgical costs in our hospital environment, there is no doubt that in all European countries we have used an increasing number of resources for the medical treatment in the more and more advanced intensive care units.

Is this of benefit to the patients? From a Swedish study Sundbärg and coworkers[4] discussed the costs of their neurosurgical intensive care units. Sundbärg compared the costs in two time periods, one from 1977 to 1978 and one from 1983 to 1984 (Table 3).

During the first period the conventional medical intensive care treatment was given for all patients, whereas during the second period advanced intensive care was used including intracranial pressure monitoring, respirator treatment, barbiturate coma etc. Although the figures cannot be exactly compared – as this was not a prospective study – it must be noted that the referral area was the same and that the treatment of the patients in each category was the same. Based on the Glasgow Coma Outcome Scale the patients were divided in good – moderate – severe– vegetative– and dead states (Table 3). The hospital costs were based on the socalled Crize index, an economical index developed by the faculty of economics of the University of Lund[1]. I have revised these official Swedish figures to German marks (DM) of 1990, adding the inflation rate in Sweden and the rate of national interests since 1977 (Table 3). In the first part of the study the mean cost per patient treated was 19.161 DM whereas it rose to 27.948 DM per patient in the second period with modern intensive care treatment. This rise of 48% must give a thrill to any good administrator or politician leading to immediate reduction of the number of patients treated in the department to reduce the budget. If we however look into what happened to the patient cared for and combine the good and moderate recoveries we find to our surprise that the total costs per good survivor in the two groups are identical. In the first time period it was 35.651 DM per patient and in the second period

Table 3. *Costs of Neurosurgical Intensive Care Units (modified from G. Sundbärg, 1988)*

Outcome GCS	1977–1978			1983–1984		
	No.	Total costs	Cost pr. patient	No.	Total costs	Cost pr. patient
Good	20	424.682	21.234	44	1.107.412	25.168
Moderate	10	203.468	20.347	13	436.079	33.545
Severe	4	151.615	37.904	6	344.016	57.336
Vegetative	2	163.453	81.727	5	219.232	43.846
Dead	31	340.455	10.982	19	324.694	17.089
Total	67	1.283.773	19.161	87	2.431.443	27.984

All costs in DM.

35.757 DM per patient. Therefore we as doctors must aim at changing the discussion of direct costs to the problem of costs related to the quality of life. This is an obligation for us as medical doctors and this fact is surprisingly not often used when debating economics of medical treatment.

Starting with social costs several different economic models have been developed. The one mainly used so far is the Human Capital Theory, whereby the use of resources are based on socalled direct costs. As an example: the doctor's fees, equipment price in hospital, wages etc. At the same time the indirect loss of resources for society are estimated such as the loss of active production by the injured worker etc. Finally is included the transferance of resources from active persons in society to the nonactive deceased patients in form of disablement pensions etc. Combining these factors we end up according to the Human Capital Theory with the price or the cost of our treatment[5]. The major problem with this theory is how the loss of resources is defined? What is "the price" of a house wife? According to the Human Capital Theory it is zero! In recent more modern studies the Theory of Willingness to Pay as a cost/benefit analysis has been introduced based on the socalled Welfare Economy[5]. The general Welfare Economy of a society includes advanges and disadvantages determined by changes of the individual person's welfare. In this theory it is the individual person and not the society alone that is the starting point for the analysis. It is the individual citizen's estimation of benefits and costs, that are mandatory, and these are all made on the individual citizen's willingness to pay for the change. If we e.g. want to involve ourselves in a prevention project estimating on reducing the number of traffic accidents by 30% – this project with cost money. We must pay to rebuild roads, increased police supervision, make bridges safer etc. These moneys are found by a reduction of costs elsewhere e.g. among welfare of the elderly, the ordinary hospital spending or by increasing the unemployment rate. Is this acceptable? What does the individual Dane think of the reduction of risk of being killed by a traffic accident compared to that of not being able to buy a new refrigerator every second year? We know from test driving that playing heavy rock music during driving makes people up to 20% more aggressive in their driving, driving faster than they would do, if they were listening to classical music. It is obvious that our society would never accept a law that interferes with our right to play rock music during driving – there will be no willingness to make this sacrifice by the youngsters.

Another example: alcohol and driving. – In Denmark the limit is by law 0,8‰. If we tempted to reduce that to zero we will have a very severe discussion in our society. We all know that up to 25% of all traffic accidents are connected with drinking and driving with an alcohol content in the blood of over 0,8‰. We know from studies in Northern Jutland that a young mans' risk of being involved in an accident is 120 times greater when he is alcohol-intoxicated than if he is not. If we make a new law instituting driving with 0,0‰ alcohol level to prevent accidents this law would be violated by the majority of Danes. It would not be accepted – there would be *no willingness to obey this law*. However our administration in Northern Jutland understood that we could not criminalize a major part of the Danish population and instead they sent out a brochure to all youngsters informing them about accident figures and the consequence of alcohol intoxication. It was a smart brochure – a tape recording with modern music and a text concerning drunk driving including a pools coupon which could be sent in whereby those who guessed right would receive a prize and some gifts. The campaign started in 1988 and immediately the number of accidents dropped and within 8 months we had in our part of the country 30% less traffic accidents among this age group than anticipated. This is an example of an acceptable project! Another important thing is when comparing accident studies, whether we use a prevalence – or an incidence method. The incidence method relates traffic accidents to the time when the costs related to the incidence starts. In other words, when the accidents happens. All costs related to specific accidents although showing in the coming years are added as shown in Table 4.

Costs related to accident A 1 = costs C 1/1 in 1988 and cost C 2/1 in 1989 is thus added in an incidence study. In a prevalence study it is only the costs in the same year that are being used. It is demonstrated in Table 4 how the differences of calculation will highly influence the apparent costs to society at a specific time. Comparison among studies are therefore related to which type of economic method is being used, a thing that is not always made clear. The prevalence study is excellent for comparing immediate economic results of a campaign on existing treatment, whereas the incidence study is more suited for a priority discussion.

Many models of economic estimation or costs within society have been found in the literature of National Economics[5]. Based on Danish studies the relative distribution among cost groups related to traffic accidents are seen in Table 5.

In other words the costs of repairing damaged materials, cars, wall, roads etc. including insurance costs

Table 4. *Calculation of Accidents Costs by Using Prevalence and Incidence Method*

A_1	C_1^1	C_1^2	A_2	C_2^1	C_2^2	A_3	C_3^1	C_3^2
1988			1989			1990		

	Prevalence	Incidence
Costs 1988	C_1^1	$C_1^1 + C_1^2$
Costs 1989	$C_1^2 + C_2^1 + C_2^2$	$C_2^1 + C_2^2 + C_3^1 + C_3^2$
Costs 1990	$C_3^1 + C_3^2$	0

For methods explanation see text. Costs are represented by (C) and Accidents by (A). First accident A_1; Second A_2; etc. C_1^1– First cost of the first accident; C_2^1 – the second cost of the first accident. Cost on the second year, etc.

Table 5. *Relative Distribution Among Cost-Groups*

Material	68,91%
Productionloss	23,79%
Hospital	6,73%
Emergency transportation	0,43%

Table 6. *Deaths Related to Production Loss (in Denmark)*

Males	
Car	85.757.300 DM
MC	42.064.400 DM
Bike	9.902.000 DM
Ped	12.787.200 DM
Total	150.510.900 DM
Total females	31.736.700 DM

Table 7. *Costs Related with Traffic Accidents in Denmark 1990*

Police; emergency transportation	9 million DM
Hospital	116 million DM
Production-loss	407 million DM
Material	1.184 million DM
Total cost Denmark	1.715 million DM

covered up to 68,91% of all costs related to the accident. The loss of production is 23,79% whereas the hospital costs are only 6,73% of all costs to society. Transportation including helicopter services will only cover roughly 0,43%–0,50%. In other words – medical doctors involved in discussions of economics always relate their influence to hospital costs and these including transportation are only 7% of the costs to society! This is another major reason why MD's must be involved in economic discussions in the future when priorities are being decided for the local community.

In Table 6 I have estimated the loss of production among all groups of males related to car accidents. Among those who die it is estimated to be 85 million DM, for motorcycles 42 million DM, for bikes 9 million DM and for pedestrians 12,7 million DM, a total of 150 million DM per year. The same figure for females are 31,7 million DM per year. If we estimate the loss of production related to *all traffic accidents* (not only car accidents) in Denmark it will be around 407 million DM in 1990. For loss of material it will be 1.100 million DM, for hospital costs 116 million DM and for police and emergency transportation 9 million DM, a total of 1,715 million DM per year in Denmark in 1990 (Table 7).

In conclusion it must be emphasized that the majority of our statistics are not valid for a sufficient discussion of economics and priorities. The medical profession must be involved in feeding the computers. Incidence studies will be a very important tool for the future.

References

1. Accident report (1985), Northern Jutland county
2. Carlsson S et al (1973) Epidemiology of head injuries. Conference Proceedings. International Conference on the Biokinetics of Impacts, Amsterdam, June 26–27
3. Economische Schade Ten Gevolge Van Verkeersonveiligheid, R-84-10, Ir. F. C. Flury, Leidschendam, 1984. Stichting Wetenschappelijk Onderzoek Verkeersveiligheid SWOW
4. Sundbärg G (1988) Neurosurgical intensive care and the management of severe head injuries. Thesis. Student Litterature, Lund
5. Trafikuheldsomkostninger (traffic accident costs). Rådet for trafiksikkerhedsforsking, ØSA, Vejdirektoratet, and laboratoriet for samfundsmedicinsk og sundhedsøkonomisk forsking, Odense University, 1983, Denmark

Correspondence: Jens Haase, M.D., Department of Neurosurgery, Aalborg Hospital, 9100 Aalborg, Denmark.

Subject Index